CONTEXTUAL FAMILY HEALTH

This book provides readers with a compelling case for the inclusion of contextual therapy in comprehensive healthcare settings by presenting its applications to individual and family health across the lifespan. Part I gives an overview of contextual therapy, including case conceptualization, assessment, intervention, and supervision. Part II provides specific recommendations for incorporating contextual therapy in diverse and multi-disciplinary settings. Case studies illustrate how concepts such as justice, loyalty, and balanced giving and receiving influence families' adjustment to chronic illnesses and mental health disorders. Accounting for the trend toward increased collaboration between providers in traditional mental health and medical settings, this book will empower clinicians to expand their current range of assessment methods, intervention techniques, and supervision experiences.

Alexandra E. Schmidt Hulst, PhD, LMFT, serves as an integrated behavioral health advisor at Rocky Mountain Health Plans. She uses her systemic training and clinical experience to coach healthcare teams in developing and implementing strategies to support team-based, comprehensive primary care.

D. Scott Sibley, PhD, LMFT, CFLE, is an Assistant Professor in Human Development and Family Sciences at Northern Illinois University. He researches commitment in couple relationships and romantic relationship formation, and operates a small private practice.

CONTEXTUAL THERAPY FOR FAMILY HEALTH

CLINICAL APPLICATIONS

**Alexandra E. Schmidt Hulst
and D. Scott Sibley**

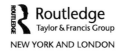

Routledge
Taylor & Francis Group

NEW YORK AND LONDON

First published 2019
by Routledge
711 Third Avenue, New York, NY 10017

and by Routledge
2 Park Square, Milton Park, Abingdon, Oxon, OX14 4RN

Routledge is an imprint of the Taylor & Francis Group, an informa business

Library of Congress Cataloging-in-Publication Data
A catalog record for this title has been requested

ISBN: 978-1-138-68482-9 (hbk)
ISBN: 978-1-138-68483-6 (pbk)
ISBN: 978-1-315-54362-8 (ebk)

Typeset in New Baskerville
by Keystroke, Neville Lodge, Tettenhall, Wolverhampton

For my grandparents, Richard and Shirley Uhrik, who have modeled enduring love and quiet, humble perseverance.

Alex Schmidt Hulst

For my students who inspire me to have the courage to research and teach about families.

D. Scott Sibley

Contents

Acknowledgments

Alex Schmidt Hulst

As Albert Schweitzer wrote, "At times our own light goes out and is rekindled by a spark from another person. Each of us has cause to think with deep gratitude of those who have lighted the flame within us." These words inspire me to remember the countless people to whom I owe deep appreciation for supporting me in personal and professional growth, both during moments of discouragement and uncertainty and moments of celebration and joy.

I am fortunate to be surrounded by an excellent tribe of other systemic thinkers and family therapists. I have had many wonderful teachers and mentors who graciously taught me the privilege of diving into the depths of joys and suffering that families experience. My identity as a clinician has been shaped by wise, humble guides such as Glen Jennings, Mary Sue Green, Connie Cornwell, Nicole Springer, Randall Reitz, and Mike Olson. Countless other therapist colleagues have inspired me with their insightful creativity, including Rola Aamar, Ashlee Miller, Jeff Crane, Cody Heath, and Cammy Froude. Thank you for the countless hours of introspection and reflection and for emboldening me with courage when I needed it.

I offer great thanksgiving for my beautifully messy, loving family—my parents, my brother, grandparents, and countless aunts and uncles and cousins. You taught me that illness is not confined to the realm of things that are scary and sorrowful and that illness can lead to opportunities for meaningful connection and unity. Thank you, thank you, thank you for your selfless sacrifices, words of reassurance, and wisdom.

To Josh, a true partner and ally in all life's adventures: I am so grateful for your uplifting words of encouragement and constant patience throughout this writing process. Your humble dedication to serving your patients well inspires me and gives me hope for a healthcare system that is genuinely compassionate and life-giving in a way that extends beyond traditional medicine. And to Dutch, my loyal canine companion: thank you for endless hours of sitting patiently at my feet while I write and reminding me when it was time to take a break and play.

Finally, I offer heartfelt gratitude to the many patients and their families whom I have served over the years. I am humbled by the ways you have shared your stories, your hearts, your pain, and your hopes with me. I am thankful for the ways you challenged me and told me when I was off-track or short-sighted and worked through the feelings of "stuckness" with me. Most of all, I am honored to share some of your stories in this book so our readers can know the gracious fortitude and courage you have shown in the face of adversity. Keep pushing me to be braver and more understanding.

D. Scott Sibley

I too am greatly indebted to many individuals for their mentoring, friendship, and support over the years. These individuals have helped me become much more than I thought I was capable of becoming; to Richard Bischoff who first ignited my love for family therapy theory, and introduced me to the Contextual Therapy framework. Rich took a chance on me years ago so that I could attend the Marriage and Family Therapy Program at the University of Nebraska-Lincoln, which I am still so very thankful for. To Paul Springer whose support, patience, and persistence have helped me achieve my goals. Paul's years of guidance and friendship have simply been incredible. To Cody Hollist and Allison Reisbig for their feedback, and supervision which was instrumental in my development while I was a beginning therapist.

For Amber Vennum who is the very best mentor a student could possibly ask for. Amber is one of the most empathetic individuals that I have ever met, and has helped me work through many personal challenges and hang-ups I have personally had as a scholar. Amber especially helped me to establish my courage and determination to write and to research. I also am very appreciative of my colleagues Cameron Brown, Jared Durtschi, Brie Turns, Jonathan Kimmes, Jaimee Hartenstein, and many others who have inspired me with their friendship and encouragement. For Scott Stanley whose scholarship and mentorship has had a substantial impact on the way I conceptualize and research about couple and family relationships. Also to my colleagues at Northern Illinois University in Human Development and Family Sciences for their exceptional work with families and their continual focus on working with families systemically.

For my beautiful, supportive, patient, and ever encouraging wife KaCee whose selfless love has transformed the way I view relationships. KaCee's love and friendship has been one of the most compelling reasons I chose to teach, research, and do therapy with families in the first place. To my children Taryn, Trevor, Landon, and Carter who constantly teach me about trust, love, and loyalty, and motivate me to become the best husband and father that I can be. To my parents who have always demonstrated the importance of serving and caring for people who are struggling. Thanks to both of you for being incredibly kind, generous, supportive, and loving to me throughout my life.

Finally, to my past, present, and future therapy clients. May each of you find the happiness, contentment, stability, and success in your relationships that so many of you are searching for.

Prologue

The concepts of fairness, trust, and loyalty are intricately entwined in the lives of the individuals, couples, and families whom we serve in our clinical work. Have you ever stopped to consider how often we take these concepts for granted? There seems to be an unspoken expectation that each of us should be treated fairly, be able to trust others, and find loyalty within our deepest relationships. Yet, some of the greatest conflicts we have within our intimate relationships and in our societal context revolve around the ideas of fairness and trustworthiness.

Beyond fairness issues, humans seem to be wired for love (e.g. Tatkin, 2011) and have a profound desire at their core to be cared for and to care for others in return. Among other components essential for satisfaction in couple and family relationships, love and attachment have experienced a resurgence in the therapeutic literature (e.g. Sandberg et al., 2016; Soloski et al., 2013). For instance, models such as emotionally focused therapy (Johnson, 2004) have received a great deal of attention in helping promote loving connection between partners and family members.

Overlooked by many clinicians, however, is contextual therapy. As one of the foundational models of systemic family therapy, this model was specifically designed to assist in restoring balance in relationships when the scales have been tipped away from love and trustworthiness and towards injustice, distrust, and instability. Van der Meiden, Noordegraf, and van Ewjik (2017) highlighted that contextual therapy, compared to other therapeutic models developed during the twentieth century, "stood out for connectedness and reciprocal care, offering an alternative for the unilateral emphasis on individualized problems and pathology" (p. 1). Although often disregarded by some clinicians as being too complex, we believe the contextual approach can be explained in a more accessible, intuitive way and can open a wide array of topics previously unexplored in therapy.

Some have considered the contextual approach to be on life support (Rosenberg & Sandberg, 2004), often forgotten in favor of more modern theories. We believe it would be incredibly unfortunate if this therapy model lost traction within the mental health field. To resuscitate the vision inherent in Boszormenyi-Nagy's approach to contextual therapy, there is a great need for therapists who can skillfully and creatively bring modern relevance to this model. This revival includes the fresh application of contextual therapy within the context of collaborative healthcare addressing needs across the biopsychosocial continuum of health.

We offer this book to readers so you may acquaint or reacquaint yourself with the contextual therapy approach and determine how best to integrate these concepts into your work with patients (the word "clients" will also be used interchangeably throughout this book). Our goal is to inspire new learners to weave selected contextual therapy concepts into your current clinical work, or if this is already your preferred approach to counseling and therapy, to further refine your skills in working with individuals, couples, and families and apply this model to families affected by a variety of health-related issues.

THE CONTEXTUAL APPEAL

Throughout history, fairness has emerged as a critical determinant of major political decisions. Mentions of fairness and justice can be found in ancient Roman laws, collections of letters written by Abraham Lincoln, modern policies concerning equal and adequate pay in the workplace, and countless decisional statements provided by judges in court cases. On a smaller level, fairness seems to be entwined in the politics of everyday family life. Young siblings often quarrel over whose turn it is to put away the dishes, couples argue about whether to defer to the other partner's preference of how to spend date night or holidays, and all individuals must grapple at some point with the fairness of a mortal life that inevitably includes times of health and times of illness.

Why does fairness seem to be so central to the decision-making process? Whether we consider decisions that are extraordinarily life-changing for a large group of people or part of the fabric of ordinary life, fairness provides a measuring stick for what seems right and what seems wrong in many difficult decisions. Difficulties arise when one person's measurement of fairness doesn't match up with another person's assessment. Far from being an American phenomenon born out of greed or individualism run rampant, we propose that human beings are naturally inclined to note contrasts between what seems just and what seems unjust. Fairness is not a luxury topping of the highest quality relationships, but a basic ingredient that is necessary for any sort of sustainability in relationships.

People yearn for relationships that seem fair and balanced, and this type of justice keeps relationships from crumbling during life's most heart-wrenching challenges. This is the basic premise of contextual therapy: people crave a way to make sense of the world and relationships in a way that builds up trust and loyalty with those with whom they are most intimate. Experiences impacting trust and loyalty generate expectations about fairness and justice within relationships, and these general expectations influence adjustment to specific dilemmas. As we'll discover throughout this book, contextual therapy is a model that accounts for both I and We factors that are part of the human experience and influence how individuals and families maintain wellness and cope with health problems over time.

MAKING THE CASE FOR INCLUSION IN MEDICINE

How do perceptions of fairness and equity influence matters of health? On a larger social level, socioeconomic status affects individuals' access to medical services, ability to afford treatment, and health literacy in comprehending complex medical decisions. Within family systems, expectations about fairness guide how families equitably (or not so equitably) divide responsibilities for emotional, financial, and physical care management. Throughout the course of illness, individuals may ponder existential questions about the meaning of suffering, pain, and discomfort. Each of these components can be addressed by medical family therapists and clinicians from various other disciplines who work within the healthcare field.

As we are continually confronted with the complexity of offering comprehensive healthcare, the modern American medical system thrives when there is successful collaboration between professionals who address multifaceted aspects of health. Collaborative teams in healthcare often include medical providers, nurses, medical assistants, dieticians, behavioral health specialists, care managers, and more. In the contextual framework, each of these professionals has an important job in addressing individual and relational factors along the biopsychosocial continuum of health. Effective, efficient, and responsible healthcare provision cannot solely focus on biomedical care, nor can it ignore the influence of psychological and social factors on preferences for treatment, adherence to medical recommendations, and health outcomes.

During times of illness, individuals and families ask many questions borne out of pain, suffering, confusion, and desperation. In this book, we propose that contextual therapy provides an essential framework for grappling with these difficult questions. Far from providing a set of trite, ready-made answers, contextual therapy presents a lens to understand patients and families' struggles with caregiving responsibilities, fears about burdening others, and hesitation to accept change or offer forgiveness for previous injustices. Contextual therapy is not the only way, but it provides a powerful shift in the way we characterize distress exhibited by families in exam rooms, hospital rooms, and outpatient therapy rooms as they cope with some of the most challenging illnesses of our time.

UNIQUE CONTRIBUTIONS OF CONTEXTUAL THERAPY

One of the primary goals of this book is to highlight specific ways that the contextual approach is unique and offers innovative avenues into conversations, creating solutions that differ from those offered by other models of systemic therapy. Within medical settings, some of the most common therapy models include cognitive behavioral therapy, motivational interviewing, acceptance and commitment therapy, narrative therapy, and solution-focused therapy. Although these models provide a powerful means of helping patients work towards health, none of them are inherently relational in nature, meaning that they do not highlight a specific emphasis on the influence of social relationships on health.

Furthermore, none of these models are intergenerational and explicitly acknowledge the role of relationship patterns across multiple generations of a family. None of these models are considered foundational models of systemic family therapy. Finally, none of these models explicitly address the elements of trustworthiness and fairness within relationships. Although these models have undeniable benefits within health management, we believe that more significant healing can be achieved with an integrated approach that accounts for the role of intergenerational family processes.

Contextual therapy is one such integrative clinical approach. In fact, we believe that one of the most useful aspects of contextual therapy is its versatility. It can be used as a primary model of therapy or integrated with other therapeutic models (e.g., Lyness, 2003; Schmidt Hulst, 2019). It can be used to treat relational issues commonly presented in couple or family therapy (e.g., Hargrave & Pfitzer, 2003; Hibbs, 2010) or for specific mental health diagnoses (Sibley, Schmidt, & Kimmes, 2015). Despite some therapists' hesitation about the accessibility of contextual therapy, Goldenthal (1993) explained:

> It is difficult to find an experienced therapist who would argue with the notion that knowledge of a person's past and present family relationships is crucial to understanding and helping the person, or one who would deny that the issues of loyalty and fairness are central to life and to close relationships. (p. xiii)

As we will discover throughout this book, the foundational concepts of contextual therapy can be applied in a wide variety of settings where couples and families seek services in managing biomedical and psychosocial health. Even if you do not personally identify as a contextual therapist in training or in practice, we believe including contextual elements in your work has the potential to create exciting new insights in your clinical work with your clients and patients.

COMMON MISUNDERSTANDINGS

Due to some common misunderstandings about contextual therapy, some clinicians may find themselves opposed to practicing therapy guided by this model. In this book, we hope to demystify the contextual approach to therapy and provide clinicians with a more complete perception of this model's unique offerings to helping families trend towards health and wellness. For instance, a common misconception is that the therapist defines what is fair. In reality, the contextual therapist's job is to help the family define what fits within their cultural and familial values and goals for meeting all members' needs. This sense of autonomy for patients to determine what is fair and balanced within their relationships is crucial. Some individuals mistake this balance of giving and receiving as a quid pro quo arrangement, but it is more accurate to consider the process of building trustworthiness and finding balance as longitudinal and occurring throughout the course of a single relationship as well as between multiple generations within a family.

Another common misunderstanding is that contextual therapy is meant to promote insight into injustices. Contextual therapy is, in fact, a therapy designed to increase insight and personal understanding about why injustices have occurred. However, it is also true that accountable action of some kind is essential to restore relational ethics. This focus on reparative action cannot be overlooked.

Finally, some clinicians may be discouraged about the contextual approach if they find the concepts elusive or vaguely defined and struggle to craft contextually based interventions based upon a rich, dense theory. However, we propose a more productive focus on application instead of the underlying theory itself. The tenets of contextual therapy were created in order to enhance clinicians' abilities to address fairness and the natural balance of giving and taking within intimate relationships. As clinicians practice skillfully addressing unspoken expectations and needs within relationships, these concepts can be immensely powerful in shifting family interactions towards fulfillment and biopsychosocial health.

DEEPENING ROOTS AND GROWING TO NEW HEIGHTS

This book is not a radical reinvention of Boszormenyi-Nagy's (1979) original conceptualization of contextual therapy, nor is it a critique of previous contextual writers' work. Rather, we are deeply appreciative of the ways in which authors such as Goldenthal (1993), Hargrave and Pfitzer (2003), and Hibbs (2010) have woven together contextual concepts and used modern clinical examples to clarify abstract concepts like justice, fairness, and loyalty. Recent articles by Sude and Gambrel (2017) and van der Meiden, Noordegraf, and van Ewjik (2017) propose clear applications of contextual therapy by elucidating ways in which a contextual framework can be used to craft clinical interventions and train clinicians, through defining clear interventions for clinical work and the training of therapists. These contextual writers have crafted an important foundation for this book, which presents a specific context where this model can be applied: multidisciplinary healthcare promoting health and wellness in individuals and families.

If we are not scheming a revolution, what are we doing with this literary endeavor? We like to think of this as more of a renaissance, a bridge between a time when contextual therapy stood at the fringes of family therapy and a time when contextual therapy will be deeply appreciated for its value in answering questions not addressed by other therapy models. It is another voice in helping families make sense out of tragedy and difficulty, finding healing in each other. We hope that this book will inspire clinical educators to teach this model earnestly, concisely, and clearly in graduate training programs for mental health professionals, instead of being dismissed for being outdated or abstruse. We also hope this book fosters conversations between clinicians that honor contextual therapy as equal in value to existing models of therapy commonly used to frame interventions within the medical system. We hope this energy ignites and spreads from those who consider themselves family therapists to those who identify as other care team members such as physicians, nurses, and care managers and are seeking a framework to make sense of family needs.

I (ASH) remember when I learned about this model in my first semester of graduate school. We had a guest lecturer who compared the balance of giving and taking, so essential in contextual therapy, to acrobatic partnered yoga. Balance, trust, and full commitment keep each partner safe in this entrancing, strengthening activity, and the same holds true for our most intimate relationships in families and in couples. As we learned about constructs such as balanced giving and receiving, trustworthiness, and loyalty, I felt something resonate deep within me. I found a way to make sense of my expectations, hopes, and disappointments in my own relationships. I had far more questions than answers about this model, and this curiosity helped me stay hungry enough to read the original writings of Boszormenyi-Nagy. Though dense and philosophical, I kept returning to his words as I learned how to apply this model to therapy I conducted with individuals and their families, all at various points along the health spectrum.

Over time, I have witnessed this model being used as a catalyst for change and healing within families, even when physical healing from an illness is impossible. I am often amused by how core concepts—trust, fairness, loyalty—can simultaneously seem incredibly simple yet impossibly complex. This model, along with others in my clinical repertoire, has been a faithful guide for me to look for the core of what nourishes trustworthiness and flexibility in families facing heath crises. It is our hope that you, too, will remain open and curious about these concepts and learn how to intertwine them in your conversations with individuals, couples, and families, wherever you may find them in their journey with health and illness.

WHAT TO EXPECT FROM THIS BOOK

Just as we believe honest conversations about expectations are important for personal relationships, we also wish to provide you with clear guidelines about what you can expect to learn through this book. In this book, we will not give a lengthy, detailed description of the underlying theory of contextual therapy. Other authors have dedicated entire books to this, and we will only focus on explaining key concepts that will be relevant to the rest of the book. In Part I, we will provide a brief orientation to the theoretical underpinnings of essential skills in contextual therapy. This will include case conceptualization, assessment, intervention, and supervision.

Once we have established this foundation, we will move on to Part II, which will focus on specific applications of contextual therapy in family health. We will provide recommendations for how to incorporate relevant contextual constructs and design interventions tailored to various settings, including brief interventions within primary care, brief interventions during inpatient hospitalization, more traditional outpatient psychotherapy models, and patient and family support groups. Throughout this section, we will use case studies to differentiate between the unique needs of families with various types of biomedical and mental health illnesses. It is important for us to note that these cases are based upon real client families with whom we have worked over the years, but important details including names, ages, medical details, and parts of the story have been changed to protect clients' anonymity while preserving the overall quality of therapeutic interactions. It is our hope that you will find these case studies helpful in developing your own personal style of putting this model into action. Let us begin.

REFERENCES

Boszormenyi-Nagy, I. (1979). Contextual therapy: Therapeutic leverages in mobilizing trust. Report 2 Unit IV. *The American Family*. Philadelphia: The Continuing Education Service of Smith Kline and French Laboratories. Reprinted in R. J. Green and J. L. Framo (Eds.), *Family therapy: Major contributions* (pp. 393–416). New York, International Universities Press (1981).

Goldenthal, P. (1993). *Contextual family therapy: Assessment and intervention procedures*. Sarasota, FL: Professional Resource Press.

Hargrave, T. D. & Pfitzer, P. F. (2003). *The new contextual therapy: Guiding the power of give and take*. New York, NY: Routledge.

Hibbs, B. J. (2010). *Try to see it my way: Being fair in love and marriage*. New York, NY: Penguin.

Johnson, S. M. (2004). *The practice of emotionally focused couple therapy: Creating connection*. New York: Brunner-Routledge.

Lyness, K. P. (2003). Extending emotionally focused therapy for couples to the contextual realm: Emotionally focused contextual therapy. *Journal of Couple and Relationship Therapy, 2*(4), 19–32. doi:10.1300/J398v02n04_02

Rosenberg, T. E. & Sandberg, J. G. (2004). The new contextual therapy: Guiding the power of give and take. *Journal of Marital and Family Therapy, 30*(3), 389–390.

Sandberg, J. G., Novak, J. R., Davis, S. Y., & Busby, D. M. (2016). The brief accessibility, responsiveness, and engagement scale: A tool for measuring attachment behaviors in clinical couples. *Journal of Marital and Family Therapy, 42*(1), 106–122.

Schmidt Hulst, A. E. (2019, In Press). Helping families heal through the death of a parent: An integration of contextual therapy and emotionally focused family therapy. *OMEGA – Journal of Death and Dying.*

Sibley, D. S., Schmidt, A. E., & Kimmes, J. G. (2015). Applying a contextual therapy framework to treat panic disorder: A case study. *Journal of Family Psychotherapy, 24*(4), 299–317.

Soloski, K., Pavkov, T., Sweeney, K., & Wetchler, J. (2013). The social construction of love through intergenerational processes. *Contemporary Family Therapy: An International Journal, 35*(4), 773–792. doi:10.1007/s10591-013-9247-5

Sude, M. E. & Gambrel, L. E. (2017). A contextual therapy framework for MFT educators: Facilitating trustworthy asymmetrical training relationships. *Journal of Marital and Family Therapy, 43*(4), 617–630.

Tatkin, S. (2011). *Wired for love: How understanding your partner's brain and attachment style can help you defuse conflict and build a secure relationship.* Oakland, CA: New Harbinger Publications.

van der Meiden, J., Noordegraf, M., & van Ewjik, H. (2017). Applying the paradigm of relational ethics into contextual therapy. Analyzing the practice of Boszormenyi-Nagy. *Journal of Marital and Family Therapy.* doi: 10.1111/jmft.12262

AN ORIENTATION TO CONTEXTUAL THEORY AND SKILLS

Chapter 1

The Theory Behind the Practice

Before learning how to use a set of tools, it is important to know what the tools are used for and how they address a problem. Although the current system of healthcare includes many treatments and techniques to improve patients' health, we propose that contextual therapy offers a unique array of tools to promote healing in a variety of dimensions. Before we can learn how to use them, however, we need to develop a rationale for why and when contextual therapy interventions could be included as part of comprehensive healthcare.

IN DEFENSE OF ASSUMPTIONS

By definition, assumptions are expectations that are accepted to be true without having proof. These suppositions serve as the foundation for a set of beliefs that guide the way we think, behave, and feel. Although problems arise when we adhere too strongly to our assumptions without exploring alternative ideas, equally serious problems emerge when we don't recognize the existence of our assumptions and how those impact our life and the lives of those around us. As the author and biochemist Isaac Asimov (n.d.) wisely reminded, "Your assumptions are your windows on the world. Scrub them off every once in a while, or the light won't come in." Notice that he did not say to get rid of all your assumptions, but to be aware of them and to consider clarifying and refining your perspective every so often so you are seeing with clearer vision.

According to Boszormenyi-Nagy and Krasner (1986), the foundation of contextual therapy is formed by two core assumptions. First, the model assumes that the consequences of any one person's decisions or actions affect the lives of all those who are connected with him or her. This conviction places this model of individual, couple, and family therapy squarely within the realm of models grounded in general systems theory, which acknowledge that a change in any one part of a system inevitably reverberates throughout the rest of the system. In other words, we do not live our lives in a vacuum. Rather, clinicians guided by a contextual framework recognize how patterns and shifts in various systems, both large and small, influence individuals' unique experiences and forever alter that system as a whole.

For example, the diagnosis of a chronic illness such as diabetes impacts other people in that person's social network, including family members, coworkers, and friends. Likewise, a decision made by an insurance company about which medications will be covered trickles down to impact the very individuals who receive benefits from that insurance provider. The insurance system also intersects with other social and environmental systems influencing individuals' experiences within the healthcare system. These systems, whether individual families or complex healthcare systems, are composed of more than just a set of objects or individuals (Gray, Duhl, & Rizzo, 1969). Rather, a comprehensive understanding of these systems accounts for both (1) individual characteristics of those who make up the system and (2) the inter-relationships between individual patients, family members, healthcare providers, healthcare policy decision-makers, and more.

The second assumption, according to Boszormenyi-Nagy and Krasner (1986), is that satisfying, fulfilling relationships include responsible consideration of and accountability for other people within the relationships we form. In other words, contextual therapy proposes that, contrary to popular belief, we are, in fact, accountable for how our decisions affect others. In the contextual view, responsibility for how we affect others is beneficial for their well-being, as well as for our own. Boszormenyi-Nagy and Krasner (1986) wrote, "Context implies consequences that flow from person to person, from generation to generation, and from one system to its successive system" (p. 8). As system members and individuals, we are not immune from acknowledging the ripple effects of our actions. Our relationships have significance in past, present, and future interconnectedness, regardless of whether members maintain active contact or not.

Research supports this assumption. The 75-year long Grant Study, run by Harvard University, demonstrated a crucial ingredient for a healthy, satisfying life: fulfilling intimate relationships with others (Itkowitz, 2016). Dr. Robert Waldinger, the current director of the study, has described the health benefits of rich intimate relationships by saying, "Good, close relationships seem to buffer us from some of the slings and arrows of getting old." At its core, this second assumption of contextual therapy reminds us as clinicians that relationships are significant for every single patient. For some readers, this may seem intuitive, and for others, unfamiliar.

How might your own practice change if you were to assume that, no matter how close or estranged, every family member of your patients is invaluably important to understanding how best to keep them healthy? What if you were to assume that encouraging your patients to consider how they affect others around them is good for their health? Unfortunately, we often accept too quickly and change the subject when a patient says, "I have not spoken to my mother in 5 years, and I do not want to talk about it" or "It does not really matter what I do. My husband does not care anyways." Contextual therapy beckons us to take a closer look at these relationships that seem strained or one-sided. The reality is that whether this patient recognizes the relationship as currently significant or not, past dynamics and meanings attached to events influence day-to-day functioning and medical decision-making. This we cannot afford to ignore.

These basic assumptions provide the foundation for core values specific to contextual therapy. As we introduced during the prologue of this book, contextual therapy clearly emphasizes concepts such as justice, fairness, loyalty, and trustworthiness. The emphasis on these values helps distinguish contextual therapy from other approaches to individual and relational psychotherapy. Here, we will briefly describe the major ideas associated with these values. Throughout the rest of this book, we will connect these key values to individual and family health experiences.

LOVE, TRUST, AND LOYALTY

One of the hallmarks of the contextual model is a recognition that throughout the course of a lifetime, each of us experiences violations of love, trust, and loyalty within relationships. We may become disappointed, jaded, or angry when our relationships do not provide the security and safety we seek. For many patients, these relational violations are at the very forefront of both physical and mental health symptom development and their decision to seek treatment in the first place. A clinician working from a contextual framework listens astutely and recognizes within the narrative presented by patients the various relational violations that have occurred and continue to occur. For clinicians guided by contextual therapy, love, trust, and loyalty are binding ingredients that preserve relationships and keep them vibrant and alive.

As a transgenerational model of family health, contextual therapy closely attends to the impact of family interactions across multiple generations on individual functionality and development of health symptoms. Relationships are divided up into two kinds: vertical relationships such as those hierarchical connections between parents and children, and horizontal relationships such as those non-hierarchical connections between siblings and romantic partners. Specific attention is paid to how patterns of behavior in vertical relationships between parents and children shape individuals' beliefs about love, trustworthiness, and loyalty. As eloquently explained by Johnson (2013), "We instinctively know that there is no other experience that will have more of an impact on our lives—our happiness and health—than our success at loving and being loved" (p. 3). We learn how to give and receive love in our families of origin, and these experiences of love (or the lack thereof) are often at the heart of many of the times of great joy and times of great pain that families experience.

For instance, some families must address parental issues manifested in the perceived favoritism of one child over another. This preference for showing love to one sibling over another can cause great friction within family relationships, and parents may struggle with determining how to give and receive love in ways that are tailored to each child's preferences and needs. This can lead to troubles between siblings, born out of hurt feelings, questions about self-worth, and dashed expectations. As explained by Boszormenyi-Nagy (1987):

> Family members may question each other's capacity for loving. One may claim that the other uses the word "love" to mean selfish receiving while he himself means giving or give-and-take of emotional exchanges. Further, people's preferences may be divided between loving and being loved—between being the subject or the object of love. (p. 85)

As we will discuss more in the next chapter, contextual clinicians hold an essential belief that relationships are most satisfactory when they allow us to be both the subject and the object of love. Although individuals may have preferences for giving or receiving care, a balance between the two is essential for sustainable growth.

Love, however, is not the whole story. Western societies may disseminate the belief that love can cure all relational ailments, but trust comprises a substantial piece of the puzzle (Hargrave & Pfitzer, 2003). For the seasoned clinician, issues revolving around trust are present within many of the conversations we have with our patients.

Although there are a myriad number of actions, big or small, that may damage individuals' experiences of love, trust, and loyalty within their family relationships, one particularly damaging example can be found in parental infidelity (Schmidt, Green, Sibley, & Prouty, 2015). Children can be haunted for years by the past decision-making of their parents, especially if they considered their parents' actions unjust and relationally unethical. For instance, Schmidt et al. (2015) found that adult children who had knowledge of their father's involvement in infidelity reported being less trusting and loyal in their own relationship with their current romantic partner. Just as we learn how to give and receive love in our families of origin, we also learn what it means to earn trust and show others that we trust them.

In some cases, discovery of infidelity can lead couples to separate or divorce with multi-systemic consequences (e.g., Amato, 2010). Regardless of parents' diligence in working to manage the fall-out, a separation and divorce inevitably change family relationships and introduce the need for significant adjustment. Research has clearly indicated that parental conflict and divorce can have a moderate impact on children and their ability to succeed in their future romantic relationships (e.g., Amato & DeBoer, 2001; Cui, Fincham, & Durtschi, 2011; Segrin, Taylor, & Altman, 2005; Rhoades et al., 2012). According to Amato (2010), "Research during the last decade continued to show that children with divorced parents, compared with children with continuously married parents, score lower on a variety of emotional, behavioral, social, health, and academic outcomes, on average" (p. 653). It is also important to note that there are protective factors—rejection sensitivity and maternal warmth, to name a couple—that help ameliorate some of the negative effects of divorce on children and adolescents and promote resiliency (Luecken, Hagan, Wolchik, Sandler, & Tein, 2017; Schaun & Vögele, 2016). As a model that places significant value on addressing violations of love, trust, and loyalty (such as those associated with infidelity and parental divorce), contextual therapy provides a framework for how to help families maintain a focus on health and well-being during times of emotional distress.

Loyalty encompasses one's sense of obligation and connection to those who have earned love and care, either by nature of their own offering of love and care or by nature of the relationship (e.g. parent and child). In a sense, it guides how individuals choose to consider, "What do I want to do?" and "What is best for us?" According to Goldenthal (1996), loyalty is not actually something that parents need to qualify for from their children. Instead, members of each generation are naturally drawn toward the desire of being loyal to previous generations.

> Contextual therapists assume that if a loyalty connection between generations is not hard-wired in, it is so universally prevalent that the potential for the development of loyalty must be so wired. We speak of being loyal as opposed to feeling loyal to emphasize that loyalty involves action, not just emotion. Loyalty is not something the parents need to earn from their offspring. (p. 74)

Even in cases in which children strive to be psychologically different than their parents, there seems to remain an innate desire to be loyal to their parental figures. Loyalty can take a variety of forms, such as maintaining family routines and traditions, following in the footsteps of a parent's career, adopting similar coping or conflict resolution strategies, or defending a parent's actions to someone expressing criticism. There are also times when a child may feel caught between two (or more) loved ones, feeling torn between relationships and how to demonstrate loyalty; not surprisingly, this pattern often emerges in families where parents are engaged in significant conflict with each other or other family members. As clinicians, we have found that it is helpful to guide clients through considering which aspects of loyalty are helpful (e.g. carrying out a favorite holiday tradition) and which may be harmful (e.g. following in the footsteps of a parent's alcoholism) rather than using a black-and-white approach with loyalty exploration.

FAIR AND SQUARE

Unique to the contextual model is the emphasis placed on fairness, which guides the flow of giving and taking that occurs within relationships. Although many people seem to have an attitude that "Life is unfair, so you should learn to accept it," our contextual lens guides us to believe that relationships can, and should be, guided by a sense of ethics steeped in a human desire for fairness. To have healthy, whole relationships, we should strive for balanced, fair justice. This means that we are accountable for a fairness that ensures that all members' needs, both for giving and receiving, are met. Although this may initially sound naïve and trite, we propose that this balanced giving and receiving is absolutely essential for having sustainable, trustworthy relationships. Van der Meiden et al. (2017) described the balance of giving and receiving as a key indicator for the quality of family life.

How do we know when a relationship is guided by fairness? What is perceived as fair differs across couples and families, which makes this a concept that is difficult to define. Perhaps the best way to describe a relationship as fair, in the contextual sense, is one that promotes a balance of giving and taking, which creates a culture of loyalty to one another and trust that all members' needs will be met over time. Fairness helps individuals to give more freely of themselves and to ask more clearly and confidently for what they need in relationships (Dankoski & Deacon, 2000).

When we speak of a balance in giving and taking, this does not mean a *quid pro quo* "I did something nice for you, now you do something nice for me" arrangement. Rather, relationships become generally balanced throughout the passage of time as both parties demonstrate a commitment to caring for each other. In the contextual framework, individuals are both obligated to demonstrate care for others and entitled to receive care from others. When we trust someone, we believe that they will "pay us back" eventually, and we don't feel the need to keep score diligently and set a deadline on when this kind deed must be repaid. Trust is maintained when others hold up their end of this unspoken deal and return love and care to us as we have shown to them.

Relationships that are fair and just adhere to the unspoken rules of relational ethics, which requires a balance in motion as members give love and care to each other and open themselves to receiving love and care from others. What may be considered fair and balanced between a parent and a young child is not the same as what is fair and balanced between a parent and an adult child; expectations shift with time, individual and relational development, and environmental changes. As Hargrave and Pfitzer (2003) described so poetically, this balance in motion within relationships is much like tightrope walking, in which you may have to shift your balance "back and forth many times in order to keep the overall balance" (p. 33). This balance of giving and taking is crucial for relationships to maintain the trust, love, and loyalty that sustains relational bonds.

As we will see when we delve into this more throughly through the later sections of this book, fairness often becomes an issue of contention during illness experiences. Patients may ask, "Why must I be sick? How is it fair that I should suffer this much?" Family members functioning as caregivers may ask, "Why do I have to do more than my fair share to take care of my mother? Shouldn't my siblings be helping me more?" Even healthcare providers struggling with burnout and compassion fatigue may question the existential fairness of suffering, which is so unavoid-able and prevalent in this demanding line of work. Added difficulties surface when enlisting the support of patients' family members who have experienced violations of love, trust, and loyalty and feel it is unfair that they should have to help care for a sick family member who has hurt them. Later sections of this book will focus on specific case examples illustrating ways in which a contextual framework can be used to concept-ualize and structure interventions to promote a restoration of fairness within families, while promoting individual health.

MAKING SENSE OF RELATIONSHIPS AND HEALTH

How exactly do our relationships influence our health? Across profes-sional fields, countless researchers have examined this question using an expansive variety of methods and theoretical lenses to frame their questions. Early contextual writers proposed a vast interweaving of relational, physical, and mental health. In acknowledging the essential need for a balance of giving and taking in relationships, Boszormenyi-Nagy (1987) warned that individuals who ignored their responsibilities to care for others were at a higher risk of developing problems such as depression, insomnia, addiction, disordered eating, sexual dysfunction, and forms of psychosomatic illness. Boszormenyi-Nagy proposed that these health problems would also be accompanied by a feeling of existential guilt since selfishness and lack of sharing of resources violate the natural order of relationships.

In addition to proposing that breakdowns in relational trust and fairness could lead to health problems, contextual founders also acknowledged the difficulties for individuals and families posed by various conditions. For example, Boszormenyi-Nagy and Krasner (1986) wrote, "Chronic illness always tests the trustworthiness of family relationships" (p. 388). Illness often necessitates a dynamic shift in the balance of giving and taking in relationships, and contextual therapy provides a powerful framework for helping families move toward health by increasing trustworthiness, restoring fairness, and demonstrating commitment and loyalty, even in the midst of physical and psychological suffering.

Some researchers have undertaken the task of finding empirical support for these theoretical assumptions. For example, Grames and colleagues (2008) conducted a nationally representative survey study to explore the associations between relational ethics, marital satisfaction, and physical and mental health outcomes. Through this study, they determined that middle-aged married adults who reported less trustworthiness, perceived fairness, and loyalty in their marriages and families of origin were more likely to report a diagnosis of health problems such as depression, anxiety, alcohol abuse, cardiac disease, and diabetes. This study showed that physical health is linked with relational health, supporting the theory underlying Boszormenyi-Nagy's claims.

WHOSE SHOW IS THIS?

As a model with a strong commitment to restoring fairness and an astute awareness of social context, contextual therapy is well suited to help couples, parents and children, and siblings during times when giving and taking has become imbalanced within relationships. The contextual model has significant utility in helping to amplify the voices of marginalized members who have experienced injustice but are inadequately acknowledged or even overtly silenced. As highlighted by feminist therapists Dankoski and Deacon (2000), "Those with more power may deem an arrangement as fair and may have more leverage in the conversations aimed at developing a consensus" (p. 56). This means that unless a clinician recognizes those with less power and acts as an advocate for social change, those with greater power within a family system will by default have more influence in defining what is fair and just.

The level of power that individuals hold within any given relationship is often linked to characteristics such as gender, race and ethnicity, age, social status, role within the family, etc. These characteristics, as well as experiences within our families of origin, influence our expectations about how to give and receive love and care. In romantic relationships, each partner enters into the relationship with expectations (often unspoken) about partners' roles and what can be considered fair. Many disappointments, grievances, and estrangements in relationships have deep roots in unmet expectations that foster a sense of injustice (e.g. Wilkie, Ferree, & Ratcliff, 1998). We like to think of relationship expectations as hidden landmines; oftentimes, you don't know it exists until you step on it and experience the explosion. When people don't feel that they're getting their needs met in relationships, power dynamics influence (1) who has the right to call attention to the injustice and (2) how balance is restored.

In addition to general relational dynamics, power is also impacted by ability status. Individuals' physical and mental abilities influence others' expectations about the level of involvement they should have in medical decision-making and the power they hold to act upon their expectations of others. Individuals with a disability, whether physical or mental, are often stigmatized and relegated to a position of lesser power, which makes it more difficult for them to advocate for themselves or other family members when injustice is occurring. Cases pertaining to debilitating medical conditions can become complicated quickly and present multiple ethical quandaries, especially when cognitive impairment is layered into diseases that also reduce physical functioning. In later chapters, we will use several case studies to illustrate specific instances of how families navigate the unclear waters of how and when patients are able to be included in decision-making.

Furthermore, ability level also affects what individuals are able to physically, emotionally, and cognitively give to others, in return for their own receiving of care. As contextual therapists, we hold a firm view that regardless of age, physical ability status, or cognitive functioning, all individuals are worthy of receiving love, care, and concern, and they are also capable of sharing love, care, and concern with others. This core belief often involves some creative ways in which clinicians and family members can identify opportunities for reciprocal giving and receiving for all members. Treatment teams operating from this contextual framework sincerely honor the value of every patient as an essential part of their family system and community, and they try to actively acknowledge ways in which patients contribute to the systems in which they live and work, regardless of their cognitive and physical capabilities.

As Dankoski and Deacon (2000) stated so well, contextual therapists should routinely analyze power dynamics affecting individuals' and families' lives, and neutrality is not to be expected in situations of abuse or dominance. Rather, a contextual framework guides clinicians to question critically how certain behavioral patterns place some family members at a disadvantage and strip them of dignity and power. Within the healthcare system, we believe that clinicians practicing within a contextual framework are ethically responsible for upholding the value of typically marginalized persons by (1) critically assessing for the influence of power dynamics on medical decision-making and relational interactions and (2) intervening when the contributions of an individual are not being adequately recognized by others. As contextual clinicians, we rely on a deeply empathetic, empowering therapeutic relationship to advocate for all family members' needs and address imbalances of power, both within families and larger systems.

FUNCTIONS OF CONTEXTUAL THERAPY

A very basic premise of contextual therapy is that balanced giving and taking has the ability to heal relationships and act as a buffer against life's most arduous difficulties. As Boszormenyi-Nagy, Grunebaum, and Ulrich (1991) wrote, "Contextual therapy converges with advances in the field of immunology, in the sense that its ultimate goal is the prevention of dysfunction and the rehabilitation and strengthening of the family's own 'immune system'—the resources of care, concern, and connection" (p. 210). The ways in which we put to work these resources of caring and connection can either boost our self-worth and our relationships with others or insidiously threaten the foundations of our own self-image and our most influential relationships.

The goals of contextual therapy are simple. Clinicians guided by a contextual perspective aim to (1) help family members understand how resources like trust, love, and loyalty are damaged by short-sighted actions that serve a single person's interest and invite injustice and imbalance in relationships and (2) create a safe environment where individuals can explore how to take action to restore balance and increase love, trust, and loyalty in their close relationships. We experience both intrapersonal and interpersonal growth when we acknowledge the need for balance in our relationships and strive to hold ourselves accountable for the ways in which our actions affect others. In the contextual view, whole-person health is attainable when we acknowledge that we have both an obligation to care for others and a right to expect love and care from others in our families and closest relationships. Rather than focus on pathology, contextual therapists emphasize how to optimize families' resources and catalyze growth for future generations (Dankoski & Deacon, 2000).

Meeting with patients and their family members can help healthcare providers obtain a more comprehensive assessment of the problem, determine how the illness impacts others in the family, create a culturally informed treatment plan, and enlist the support of the family in carrying out that plan (McDaniel, Campbell, Hepworth, & Lorenz, 2005). How might the broader goals of contextual therapy be applied to support families within the healthcare system? First, it is important for us to clarify that not all families who have an individual being treated for a medical condition need extensive therapeutic intervention, and not all patients and their families who need therapeutic intervention would be best treated using a contextual approach. Unfortunately, our experience has shown us that family-based therapeutic intervention within healthcare is sometimes reserved for families clearly in the most need of help and change. These are families that tend to exhibit extremely dysfunctional behaviors that are difficult to ignore and ultimately interfere with patients' compliance with treatment recommendations and medical providers' abilities to do their jobs.

In this book, we support the recommendations of McDaniel, Campbell, Hepworth, and Lorenz (2005) for family-oriented primary care, acknowledging the benefits of including family members in routine visits whenever the health problem is likely to have a significant impact on the family or when family members have resources to share as part of the treatment plan. Contextual interventions can be used to provide (1) assistance for families that might be readily recognized as experiencing difficulty in managing physical and mental health treatment and (2) encouragement for families who are taking actions to maintain balance and fairness despite the demands of illness. In the former case, longer and more targeted interventions may be needed to help enact significant changes and restore balance within the family system, many times after addressing some more serious symptoms of mental health disorders and adding in some stabilizing resources to promote safety and functional coping. In the latter case, briefer interventions can be used to highlight significant individual and familial strengths that promote trustworthiness and fairness; perhaps only small changes will need to be made to ensure balanced processes related to giving and taking. Later chapters will include a description of how to tailor contextual-based interventions to brief, time-limited interventions often used in medical settings.

Within traditional mental health and medical settings, outcomes and specific treatment goals vary from patient to patient. However, contextual-based interventions can generally be considered successful when patients and their families (1) reach a place of acceptance with the dynamic, ever-shifting balance of giving and taking within their specific family context, (2) are no longer significantly distressed by symptoms of depression, anxiety, and other mental health disorders, (3) engage regularly with each other to communicate needs, and (4) actively work toward restoring balance when habits shift and relational resources are damaged. When contextual therapy is used to manage health across the biopsychosocial spectrum, additional markers of success can include reduction of symptoms that occur as part of a specific disease process (e.g. hypertension, diabetes, psoriasis) and are exacerbated by stress. As we'll discuss more throughout this book, sometimes success in contextual therapy for family health means actively working to stop or slow the progression of disease, and sometimes success includes acceptance of functional limitations, inevitable mortality, and management of symptoms. No matter the expected prognosis or outcome for individuals' physical bodies, however, contextual interventions can help facilitate healing within individuals' minds, spirits, and relationships.

REFERENCES

Amato, P. R. (2010). Research on Divorce: Continuing trends and new developments. *Journal of Marriage and Family, 72*(3), 650–666.

Amato, P. R. & DeBoer, D. D. (2001). The transmission of marital instability across generations: Relationship skills or commitment to marriage? *Journal of Marriage and Family, 3*(4), 1038.

Asimov, I. (n.d.). Isaac Asimov quotes. Retrieved March 31, 2016 from www.goodreads.com/quotes/667214-your-assumptions-are-your-windows-on-the-world-scrub-them

Boszormenyi-Nagy, I. (1987). *Foundations of contextual therapy: Collected papers of Ivan Boszormenyi-Nagy, MD.* New York: Brunner/Mazel.

Boszormenyi-Nagy, I., Grunebaum, J., & Ulrich, D. (1991). Contextual therapy. In A. S. Gurman & D. P. Kniskern (Eds.), *Handbook of family therapy* (Vol. II, pp. 200–238). Bristol: Brunner/Mazel.

Boszormenyi-Nagy, I. & Krasner, B. R. (1986). *Between give and take: A clinical guide to contextual therapy.* New York, NY: Brunner/Mazel.

Cui, M., Fincham, F. D, & Durtschi, J. A. (2011). The effect of parental divorce on young adults' romantic relationship dissolution: What makes a difference? *Personal Relationships, 18*(3), 410–426.

Dankoski, M. E. & Deacon, S. A. (2000). Using a feminist lens in contextual therapy. *Family Process, 39*(1), 51–66.

Grames, H. A., Miller, R. B., Robinson, W. D., Higgins, D. J., & Hinton, W. J. (2008). A test of contextual theory: The relationship among relational ethics, marital satisfaction, health problems, and depression. *Contemporary Family Therapy, 30,* 183–198.

Goldenthal, P. (1996). *Doing contextual therapy: An integrated model for working with individuals, couples, and families.* New York: W.W. Norton.

Gray, W., Duhl, F. J., & Rizzo, N. D. (1969). General systems theory and psychiatry. Boston, MA: Little, Brown, and Company.

Hargrave, T. D. & Pfitzer, P. F. (2003). *The new contextual therapy: Guiding the power of give and take.* New York, NY: Routledge.

Itkowiz, C. (2016, March 2). Harvard researchers discovered the one thing everyone needs for happier, healthier lives. *The Washington Post.* Retrieved February 25, 2018 from ww.washingtonpost.com/news/inspired-life/wp/2016/03/02/harvard-researchers-discovered-the-one-thing-everyone-needs-for-happier-healthier-lives/

Johnson, S. M. (2013). *Love sense: The revolutionary new science of romantic relationships.* New York, NY: Little, Brown, and Company.

Luecken, L. J., Hagan, M. J., Wolchik, S. A., Sandler, I. N., & Tein, J.-Y. (2017). A longitudinal study of the effects of child-reported maternal warmth on cortisol stress response 15 years after parental divorce. *Psychosomatic Medicine, 78*(2), 163–170.

McDaniel, S. H., Campbell, T. L., Hepworth, J., & Lorenz, A. (2005). *Family-oriented primary care.* New York, NY: Springer.

Rhoades G., Stanley S., Markman H., & Ragan E. (2012). Parents' marital status, conflict, and role modeling: Links with adult romantic relationship quality. *Journal of Divorce & Remarriage, 53*(5), 348–367.

Schaun, V. K. & Vögele, C. (2016). Resilience and rejection sensitivity mediate long-term outcomes of parental divorce. *European Child and Adolescent Psychiatry, 25*(11), 1267–1269.

Schmidt, A. E., Green, M. S., Sibley, D. S., & Prouty, A. M. (2015). Effects of parental infidelity on adult children's relational ethics with their partners: A contextual perspective. *Journal of Couple and Relationship Therapy, 15*(3), 193–212.

Segrin, C., Taylor, M. E., & Altman, J. (2005). Social cognitive mediators and relational outcomes associated with parental divorce. *Journal of Social and Personal Relationships, 22*(3), 361–377.

van der Meiden, J., Noordegraf, M., & van Ewjik, H. (2017). Applying the paradigm of relational ethics into contextual therapy. Analyzing the practice of Boszormenyi-Nagy. *Journal of Marital and Family Therapy.* doi: 10.1111/jmft.12262

Wilkie, J. R., Ferree, M. M., & Ratcliff, K. S. (1998). Gender and fairness: Marital satisfaction in two-earner couples. *Journal of Marriage and Family, 60*(3), 577–594.

Chapter 2

Intertwining Individuality and Relatedness

As William James (1909) once wrote, "We are like islands in the sea, separate on the surface but connected in the deep." This reminds us of the powerful ways in which contextual therapy attends to the intersection of individual experiences within our most intimate relationships. One of the fundamental strengths of this model is that it provides some structure to help those working with patients and their families to better assess the complexities of both individual and relational versions of human experience.

The contextual framework conceptualizes human experience as being comprised of four dimensions: objectifiable facts, individual psychology, systemic interactions, and relational ethics. For readers unfamiliar with these dimensions as conceptualized within the contextual model, we will briefly describe aspects of human experience within each category. Then, we will describe how those dimensions influence individuals' expectations within couple and family relationships and how these four dimensions relate to the biopsychosocial-spiritual model of health and wellness.

FOUR DIMENSIONS OF HUMAN REALITIES

Objectifiable Facts

The first dimension of human experience pertains to objective facts, which are sometimes referenced as factual predeterminants (Boszormenyi-Nagy & Krasner, 1986). Although you may not be accustomed to labeling them as objective facts, chances are that your clinical assessment already includes attention to facts such as individuals' biological sex, gender, age, racial and ethnic background, employment status, health history, history of abuse, religious affiliation, and socioeconomic status. Facts that occur within family life—birth order of siblings, marriage, adoption, divorce, separation—are also relevant to understanding individuals' experiences throughout life. Some facts, such as puberty or parenthood or death, are related to transitions throughout individuals' life cycles.

In some cases, these factual circumstances and their consequences can be somewhat reversible, such as when a person's illness goes into remission or a family's financial situation improves enough to pull them out of poverty. Others, such as the death of a child or the terminal illness of a parent, cannot be reversed. Using a strength-based approach, clinicians operating from a contextual framework can help patients explore ways in which they can take action to transform even the most tragic facts and their consequences into experiences that build trust and a sense of committed closeness within the family.

Within family-oriented care, it is important to attend to the facts associated with all individuals within the family, not just those of the identified patient. This is a crucial point to take into consideration when implementing family-oriented care, especially in medicine where the focus is usually limited to the identified patient. Some facts may be common to all family members, while others—such as psychosomatic inclinations or educational attainment—may be unique to each member. Context matters in murky, confusing situations. For instance, parents' insistence upon rigid rules for their adolescent child and prioritizing school over all social commitments makes much more sense when you realize that the parents grew up in debilitating poverty and have struggled to make ends meet their entire lives. Acknowledgment of this fact offers resources for connection and shared values and goals instead of fuel for dissent and tension. An important distinction to make is that these facts require the attention of the clinician independently of how people make meaning out of them. Personal reactions and meaning-making are specifically addressed in the next dimension.

Individual Psychology

In the contextual framework, this second dimension attends to the mental events of each person. Individual psychology refers to a mix of various motivational mechanisms, which include instincts such as avoidance of anger, anticipated needs and expectations within relationships, learned patterns of behavior for self and others, and perceptions of reality and associated meanings (Boszormenyi-Nagy, 1981). External events, such as facts from the first dimension, are activated by the ways in which individuals perceive the situation, act, and respond to a constantly changing environment with responses from others. Two people can experience the same facts, such as when siblings grow up in the same household with parents who divorce, but their individual psychology includes the unique ways in which they process and respond to these facts.

There are many different psychological theories, ranging from psychodynamic to narrative, that attempt to explain how humans make sense of external events, formulate plans for action, and respond to others. The contextual approach does not endorse any of these particular models or create its own theory of individual psychology, which adds to its versatility in combining this framework with other lenses of human psychology. In our minds, we believe this increases the appeal for clinicians operating from a wide variety of theoretical models and having vastly different theories about humans' meaning-making processes. Although the original contextual framework has some roots in Freud's psychodynamic theories which emphasize humans' search for pleasure, the contextual model acknowledges that the capacity to sustain life and the freedom to enjoy what life has to offer also comes from contributing care to others and earning the right to be cared for by others (Boszormenyi-Nagy & Krasner, 1986). In contextual therapy, we earn entitlement to receive care from others in two ways: (1) by the very nature of the relationship, such as when parents have an inherent responsibility to demonstrate care for their children and (2) by showing care to others that should then be repaid in order to maintain relational justice.

Acknowledging the interconnectedness of thoughts and feelings, individual psychology can also include individuals' unique emotional experiences. Boszormenyi-Nagy and Krasner (1986) called attention to the ways in which emotions such as joy, sorrow, frustration, anger, and guilt are closely linked to whether relationships are balanced or imbalanced. If people feel they are not receiving just care from others, they are likely to feel angry and exploited. On the other hand, if they are receiving a great deal of support from others without returning that care and offering appreciation, they are likely to experience a sort of existential guilt as they recognize this imbalance.

Finally, this dimension also includes an assessment of how our clients or patients construct their identities and which parts of themselves they readily present to others. One crucial element concerns how much of our individual identity we connect with our family histories, cultural experiences, and social values. For some, identity is perceived as a very individual construct, separate and unique from the ways in which they were raised. For others, individual identity becomes enmeshed within the family's identity and preferences. As many theories of human development and family functioning warn us, problems are likely to surface with either of these two extreme ways of constructing identity. Rather, contextually minded clinicians are likely to ask of their patients, "How can you develop an identity unique to yourself while also remaining loyal to your family traditions, community experiences, and cultural values?" As we will discuss in later sections of this book, individual identity can also assess for how closely individuals identify with biomedical and mental health diagnoses.

Systemic Interactions

The contextual framework specifically addresses the role of communication and interactions in relationships. As explained by Hargrave and Pfitzer (2003), systemic interactions are "the method by which the system lets members know how they are regarded and what rules and beliefs govern their interactions" (p. 47). Clinicians who incorporate a systemic framework, whether that pertains to family-oriented medicine or psychotherapy, recognize that family members' communication and behavioral patterns are essential in understanding individual and social functioning. Complex interactions can be found in any system, such as a workplace or neighborhood community, but Hargrave and Pfitzer (2003) added, "It is the family, however, where we learn the most important rules of systemic interaction" (p. 47). It is generally in our family relationships where we first observe people interacting with each other and learn how to communicate within relationships. Families provide a training ground to develop ideas about what to expect from life, how to view ourselves, and how to value the connections we have with others.

For a clinician wishing to increase his or her understanding of family relationships as they influence individual functioning, one of the best starting places is carefully observing how couples and families interact with each other during medical appointments or therapy sessions. As our experience has shown us, there are moments during work with couples or families when it becomes incredibly clear that multi-generational patterns or interactional cycles exist. For example, you may notice over the course of an appointment that whenever a husband starts raising his voice, his wife puts her hand on his knee and gives it a squeeze and tries to change the subject. In another appointment, you notice that an adolescent sighs quietly and rolls his eyes when his mom says, "I just want what's best for him, but it's fine if he makes his own choices. My mother never allowed me to disagree with her, but I'm a different kind of mom." As you give yourself permission to be more curious about what you observe, these behavioral interactions will become more easily identifiable.

Just as you can observe behavioral patterns in appointments where multiple family members are present, you can also learn to be attentive to signs of common systemic interactions when you're working with an individual patient. This is a more nuanced, still important, therapeutic undertaking. While it may feel at times that you are only receiving one perspective from an individual patient, the language and tone they use to describe interactions in their relationships can convey a lot of information. For instance, young adult patients may complain that it always feels like their parents are nagging when discussing college, marriage, and other future plans. One could simply take this at face value and conceptualize this as a normal problem at this stage of life or characterize it as familial conflict. However, a contextual framework encourages curiosity about the expectations these parents have for their young adult and how this is played out during family conversations and gatherings. Conceptualizing this experience through the contextual dimension of systemic interactions also encourages curiosity about who in the family thinks similarly about these expectations, who feels very differently, and how these expectations play out in repetitive cycles within the family. Although it requires a higher level of thinking beyond just the patient in the room with you, an observant clinician can find great reward in striving to conceptualize the perspectives of others not attending therapy but intimately engaged in the presenting problem. Families can be as much a part of the solution as they can be (part of) the problem.

Many of the patterns and cycles we find ourselves in have their roots in past experiences with family members and romantic partners. Many patterns that seem counterproductive and destructive have developed from past hurts and violations of love, trust, and loyalty within our most intimate, formative relationships. As you begin more astute clinical observations of complex interactions and build a more refined framework to make sense of what you are seeing, you may develop a sense that certain dynamics within the family are contributing to unfairness and imbalance, which leads to individual and family distress. As a clinician working with families, you can determine how you wish to help the family begin a restructuring of these destructive interactions. Although there are many methods for and nuances of doing this, one core concept of helping family members to restructure negative interactions is that this process requires the clinician to make an overt effort to create a solid working alliance with each family member (Hargrave & Pfitzer, 2003) and assess for all members' investment in creating change.

A variety of negative interactions may exist within the family system that cause substantial turmoil and suffering. As described by Hargrave and Pfitzer (2003), "In families we find power issues, emotional splitting, scapegoating, problem patterns like taking drugs or having affairs, parentification, fusion, or disengagement" (p. 55). Clinicians working from a contextual perspective fundamentally believe that they have an obligation to hold all family members accountable for their own behaviors that contribute to dysfunctional patterns within their relationship (Boszormenyi-Nagy, 1987). A defining goal of contextual therapy is to help people within relationships to be more considerate, give more freely of themselves (especially in family relationships), and communicate with others more openly about needs and desires (Goldenthal, 1996).

It is critical to remember that contextual therapy does not ask clinicians to take an expert position and define what is fair and functional and what is not; rather, clinicians must approach the family system in a respectful way that seeks to understand how the claims and interests of each member of a family are justified. In other words, contextual clinicians recognize the ways in which each family member has contributed both constructively and destructively (Hargrave & Pfitzer, 2003). Although it can be a daunting task, the job of a contextually minded clinician is to (1) identify patterns and relational interactions that help strengthen or threaten relational ethics, (2) assess for how individual actions contribute to this absence or presence of relational balance, (3) understand all individuals' needs and claims as to why they have acted in such a way, and (4) advocate for actions to restore justice, trustworthiness, and loyalty within the family system.

Relational Ethics

The final dimension seeks to capture the experience of relational ethics, a unique construct that sets apart contextual therapy from other models of systemic therapy. Relational ethics, considered to be the cornerstone of the contextual therapy approach, both supersedes and encompasses the previous three dimensions (Boszormenyi-Nagy & Krasner, 1986). Despite pressure to maintain a fast-paced working environment (especially found in today's healthcare system), a clinician working from the contextual approach must be careful not to breeze through the first three dimensions we have previously outlined, or it can become difficult to fully understand and conceptualize this fourth dimension. In other words, the nuances of relational ethics only make sense within the context of factual demographics and lived experiences, individuals' psychological states, and the dynamic interactions that occur within relationships. If a clinician does not understand these most basic aspects of human experience, it can become exceptionally challenging to provide patients with authentic empathy and validation.

Relational ethics encompasses the giving-and-taking that fundamentally occurs in all relationships. As we have begun describing throughout the beginning of this book, healthy relationships are sustained when we both give and receive in relationships and our contributions are appropriately and graciously acknowledged by others. A relationship high in relational ethics bears the fruits of trustworthiness, justice, and loyalty, which create a strong foundation of love and commitment. In relationships that are just and help to build up our individual self-worth and relational identity, we are prepared to juggle the demands of loyalty to our family identity and the seeking of personal independence. It becomes safe for us to give to others and sacrifice what we might want for ourselves because we are able to trust that our partner, parent, or sibling will do the same for us someday. This cycle of balanced giving-and-taking creates a fertile ground for loving, kind, compassionate experiences that encourage both relational and individual growth.

What happens when things don't go this smoothly? Relationships that struggle with low levels of relational ethics are characterized by poisonous reactions such as insensitivity, impatience, resentment, hostility, and contempt. When relationships become imbalanced, this injustice can lead to significant emotional strains for one or for both people within the relationship. The constant uncertainty and ambiguity of unbalanced relationships can take a terrible toll, especially if this unethical relationship is long-term and ongoing. Imbalance isn't just toxic for relationships; there can also be individual consequences. Some research has demonstrated an association between lower levels of relational ethics and more physical and mental health problems such as depression (Grames, Miller, Robinson, Higgins, & Hinton, 2008). Contextual clinicians seek to recover, rebalance, and reestablish healthy forms of functioning when they encounter individuals experiencing unfair, unloving, and untrustworthy relationships. When it is clear that patients and their families are struggling with injustice and experiences that destroy rather than build up trustworthiness, the job of the clinician is to make an intentional effort to begin rebalancing fairness in relationships by addressing the distribution of relational benefits and burdens (Boszormenyi-Nagy & Krasner, 1986). Throughout the second half of this book, we'll provide some specific case examples for what this looks like within the context of multidisciplinary, team-based healthcare.

You may be wondering, how does this influence my role as a clinician working with patients and their families? Boszormenyi-Nagy and Krasner (1986) wrote that contextual clinicians should "operate out of a conviction that all family members gain from trustworthy relationships . . . it is the therapist's task to engender a search for the visible and invisible contributions of every family member" (p. 58). This can be easier said than done; some individuals' contributions can be readily identified, but others' require a modicum of open-mindedness and creativity, especially in families in which many injustices have occurred. As you consider how this book will influence your own clinical practice, one question to keep in mind is, "How will I hold myself accountable for looking for the ways in which every one of my patients is contributing to his or her family or community, even when I have a negative personal reaction to this person?"

Understanding the complex interactions between all four dimensions is crucial for every clinician engaging in contextually based work with individuals, couples, and families. Corners cannot be skipped; each dimension must be addressed for this clinical work to provide the most effective patient care, and, we would argue, fulfilling work for practitioners themselves. As expressed by Hargrave and Pfitzer (2003), "All the dimensions are dynamic and interactive in a mutually supportive function. The four dimensions, therefore, are mutually dependent upon one another. This fact makes it difficult to articulate one dimension as being more powerful than the others" (p. 11).

Great Expectations

In our families in which we are raised, we develop a script of beliefs that are relevant to our later relationships. According to Hibbs (2009), "Your fairness model isn't formally taught, but, more powerfully, is learned through growing up in your family. Family relationships forge expectations for give-and-take that are handed down over many generations" (p. 8). Based upon how we are treated by our parents and siblings, we develop ideas about what is fair and how much we owe our family members. Through trial and error and life-shaping experiences, we painstakingly learn what feels balanced and fair to us, as well as what leads us to feel fulfilled or unfulfilled in our relationships.

Take a moment to think about expectations that influence your own relationships with your parents. Do you expect them to call you on the phone, or are you expected to be the one to make the call? How do you expect them to react when you share good news with them, or tragic news of a disappointment? How do you expect to contribute to their care as they age? How well does this match with what they might believe you should do? Our expectations shape our beliefs about what we owe others and what they owe us, and they cannot be erased and can often be difficult to re-shape. The problem lies not in their existence, but in incongruence between two people's beliefs about what should be expected.

Although expectations of parents and children are unique to each family and even within families, the contextual framework provides some basic guidelines. Parents, as guardians of young children who are physically and emotionally vulnerable, are obligated to meet their children's basic needs—such as food, shelter, and water—and provide them with clear guidance and comfort. Parents have a responsibility to care for their children, and this responsibility cannot be ignored without serious consequences for both parents and children (Boszormenyi-Nagy & Krasner, 1986). Likewise, parents can also expect their children to demonstrate care and responsibility within the family in developmentally appropriate ways. For example, a 5-year-old child could reasonably be expected to help set the table for dinner, but it would be inappropriate in the parent-child hierarchy to expect him to be his mother's primary source of emotional comfort during a period of unemployment and tension within her marriage.

The previous section of this chapter focused on how clinicians can use four dimensions to better understand the complexity of the human experience. An example from the above paragraph can illustrate how these interwoven dimensions could be used to understand the development of expectations within parent-child relationships. Dylan is a 5-year-old male, and he lives with his mother Rhonda and his father Jake. Rhonda is experiencing a recurrent episode of major depressive disorder, triggered by the recent discovery that Jake is having an affair and the recent loss of her job as a nurse. Her depression symptoms have become moderate to severe and include sleeping up to 13 hours per day, difficulty concentrating, and emotional over-eating. Jake attempts to speak to Rhonda about the affair and apologize and promise it will not happen again, but Rhonda has disengaged and treats him with stony silence. This silence has trickled down into the relationship they each have with Jake, as both parents seem disengaged and lost in their own confusion and hurt. When Rhonda stays in her room for most of the day, Dylan brings her meals in bed and tries to sing her songs to help her feel better, with limited success in brightening her mood. Dylan is currently experiencing limited supervision from his parents, and he spends hours at a time watching TV shows. He has also missed several days of school when Jake is working and Rhonda is unable to leave her room to drive him to school. When Dylan does go to school, his teacher observes that his play takes on a strong theme of him taking care of others, and when the other children don't allow him to engage in caretaking behavior, he becomes frustrated and angry. He loudly yells on the playground one day, "But it is my job to take care of you!"

In dimension one, relevant facts include Dylan's young age and the fact that Dylan lives in a home with his biological parents. In dimension two, individual psychology includes Rhonda's history of and current experience with depression and Dylan's beliefs about his role in caring for others. In dimension three, Rhonda and Jake seem locked in a pursue-withdraw cycle, and this interaction has trickled into their relationship with their son as they both have disengaged from him. Dimension four concerns the relational ethics part of the equation, influenced by all other dimensions. The contextual framework guides us to consider the ways in which problems in Rhonda and Jake's relationship have led to an imbalanced parenting strategy that places their son Dylan in the position of providing an age-inappropriate level of care and comfort. Although it is wise to encourage prosocial and kind behavior in children, Dylan feels overwhelmingly responsible for his parents' well-being and is receiving little in return. These beliefs certainly have implications for Dylan's expectations about receiving little from his parents and feeling as if it is his duty to take care of them, and we wonder how these beliefs will shape his future relationships as he evolves throughout childhood, adolescence, and into adulthood.

Just as expectations operate within parent-child relationships, these expectations can have a substantial impact on functioning within couple relationships. A healthy couple relationship requires a steady balance of give-and-take within the relationship that emphasizes fairness. As thoughtfully explained by Hibbs (2010), "Fairness is that enigmatic, critical component of an enduring, loving, happy relationship. Unromantic as it sounds, it takes fairness to sustain love . . . imbalances of fairness underlie many problems that ail relationships" (p. 5). Within a couple relationship, expectations about fairness often influence us to expect that our partner will automatically recognize how to give us as much care and comfort as we need and graciously accept what we offer to them. Although this unspoken expectation may seem natural, the early years of a relationship often include an illumination of the ways in which our expectations don't match up with those of our partner. It takes time to find a balance and rhythm. When we feel out of sync and off-balance as if we are giving far more than we are receiving, we are prone to deep feelings of loneliness, frustration, and questions about our self-worth. From the very first moments of life, humans have a deep desire to be loved and cared for; this is necessary for survival. We especially feel entitled to loving, trustworthy, and fair behavior from a person who is committed to an intimate relationship with us. Close connections with others include a lifelong series of negotiations, spoken or unspoken, about how to keep relationships balanced.

Overlapping Definitions of Human Experience

One of the beautiful things about humanity is that we can describe our experiences in many different ways, using various lenses and frameworks. The traditional biomedical model emphasizes pathology and eliminating or slowing pathological processes (McDaniel, Doherty, & Hepworth, 2014). Although this approach has its benefits, there are also many ways in which it fails to capture the complexity of treatment needed and how to explain what leads to suffering and distress for patients.

As a response to the biomedical model which focuses primarily on bodily disease processes and biomedical interventions, Engel (1977) proposed the biopsychosocial (BPS) model of healthcare. The use of the biopsychosocial approach in medical family therapy encourages clinicians to look for the "seamless web of connections among body, mind, family, and community, as well as connections between their own experiences with illness and the experiences of their patients" (McDaniel et al., p. 96). The BPS model provides a systematic framework for assessing how biological (e.g. genetic predisposition, symptoms, diagnosis, medical treatment), psychological (e.g. thoughts, feelings, state of mental health), and social (e.g. family relationships, socioeconomic status, social support systems) factors influence disease processes, health outcomes, and the delivery of healthcare (Hatala, 2013; Hodgson, Lamson, & Reese, 2007).

With the BPS approach at the core of assessment and intervention, clinicians recognize relationships (both between patients and others in their social network and between patients and providers) at the center of healthcare, elicit patients' history within a developmental and cultural life context, and create multidimensional treatment plans. Although all dimensions are relevant to patients' comprehensive health and wellness, clinical skill is needed to determine on a case-by-case basis which of these factors is most important at the time to help patients understand and work toward health. Although this may sound overwhelming for one clinician to conduct such a thorough, comprehensive assessment and structure-multifaceted interventions, the BPS approach can be found at the heart of team-based healthcare, which relies on collaboration from a multidisciplinary team in order to meet patients' diverse needs across all factors. For example, a team could include (1) medical staff such as physicians, nurses, and medical assistants who share expertise in biomedical factors influencing illness, (2) mental and behavioral health providers to help address psychological components of medical decision-making and adherence to treatment recommendations, and (3) social workers or care managers to address social factors driving health outcomes and engagement in the medical system.

Although not initially included in Engel's biopsychosocial approach, Wright, Watson, and Bell (1996) called attention to the role of spirituality in understanding patients' and families' experiences with health and illness. Beyond identification with a specific religious affiliation, the beliefs that patients and families ascribe to the causes and purpose of illness, pain, disability, and death have extraordinary implications for how they interact with the health system and what their goals of care might be. Thus, for many professionals wishing to honor the role of spirituality and meaning-making, the biopsychosocial approach was reshaped into the biopsychosocial-spiritual (BPSS) approach. To assist providers in gathering comprehensive assessment data, Hodgson, Lamson, and Reese (2007) created an interview method addressing biopsychosocial-spiritual elements of health and illness.

You may be wondering, what role does the biopsychosocial-spiritual model play in a contextual framework? The four dimensions of contextual therapy overlap in some important ways with the aspects of human experience accounted for by the BPSS model, and there are also ways in which the two frameworks strengthen each other by focusing on some different specifics. One commonality includes the fact that both frameworks account for individual and relational experiences. These are represented in the individual psychology and systemic transactions dimensions of the contextual framework, as well as in the psychological and social aspects of the BPSS model. Likewise, both approaches aim to treat the whole person, recognizing that effective healthcare manages more than just physical symptoms and diagnoses; rather, effective, satisfactory care must include an appreciation of patients' developmental and sociocultural context.

We believe that an integration of the contextual therapy framework and the biopsychosocial-spiritual model can provide a unique vision for clinicians. For example, the contextual framework does not directly recommend specific ways in which to address spirituality with patients, although one could argue for inclusion of personal beliefs in the individual psychology dimension or social engagement of religious practices in the systemic interactions dimension. However, spirituality and meaning-making are core components of the biopsychosocial-spiritual approach. For couples and families experiencing problems with health and illness, spiritual matters often underlie the stress associated with making difficult decisions and day-to-day coping. It can be difficult to come to grips with the diagnosis of a chronic or life-threatening illness, and recognizing and reinforcing spiritual resources can provide patients and families with an important avenue with which to navigate uncertainty and create meaning from suffering and loss.

Similarly, families' involvement in spiritual discussions and experiences can help create shared meaning and purpose. We see the clinician's role in these encounters as (1) providing space and autonomy for patients to define and reflect upon spiritual beliefs that help create positive coping strategies and (2) validating patients' deeply held spiritual beliefs and making connections between beliefs and patients' choices and options regarding healthcare decisions. As you may be realizing, this is not so much a matter of religion (although that can certainly be part of this assessment), as it is discussing how patients are making sense of a difficult and life-changing diagnosis. Adding in contextual elements reminds clinicians to be curious about how individuals' spiritual beliefs interact with other family members' spiritual beliefs and how those are related to their life experiences and relationships. By combining contextual therapy and the BPSS approach, the clinician has a more robust framework for remaining curious about the various ways in which spirituality influences patients' and families' journeys through health and illness.

Just as with spiritual matters, incorporating social aspects of human experience found in the BPSS model into a contextual framework results in a more comprehensive picture of human experience. There is some overlap between the third dimension of systemic interactions in contextual therapy and the social aspect of the BPSS model, but the social aspect of the BPSS model is broader and concerns people's social ties with family, friends, coworkers, neighbors, church community members, and more. There is less of a focus on deep processes embedded within these relationships and more insight gained by understanding the value of these relationships in promoting health and wellness. In the systemic interactions dimension of contextual therapy, however, there is a more nuanced exploration of cycles and processes relevant to intimate relationships such as romantic partnerships and families.

In a similar fashion, the psychological component of the BPSS model is enhanced by reflecting upon connections with the dimension of relational ethics in contextual therapy. Individuals' psychological health, including thoughts, feelings, and behaviors, are intricately tied to experiences that either promote or threaten trust, fairness, and loyalty. These constructs, not explicitly accounted for in the BPSS model, are included as cornerstones in the contextual framework, adding to a multi-faceted assessment of how individuals maintain mental and emotional health within relationships with others. In the next chapter, we will discuss tips for addressing key components of the BPSS model and contextual therapy framework through comprehensive, ongoing assessment and treatment planning.

REFERENCES

Boszormenyi-Nagy, I. (1981). Contextual therapy: Therapeutic leverages in mobilizing trust. In R. J. Green & J. L. Framo (Eds.), *Family therapy: Major contributions* (pp. 393–416). New York, NY: International Universities Press.

Boszormenyi-Nagy, I. (1987). *Foundations of contextual therapy: Collected papers of Ivan Boszormenyi-Nagy, MD.* New York: Brunner/Mazel.

Boszormenyi-Nagy, I. & Krasner, B. R. (1986). Between give and take: A clinical guide to contextual therapy. New York, NY: Brunner/Mazel.

Engel, G. L. (1977). The need for a new medical model: A challenge for biomedicine. *Science, 196*, 129–136.

Goldenthal, P. (1996). *Doing contextual therapy: An integrated model for working with individuals, couples, and families.* New York: W.W. Norton.

Grames, H. A., Miller, R. B., Robinson, W. D., Higgins, D. J., & Hinton, W. J. (2008). A test of contextual theory: The relationship among relational ethics, marital satisfaction, health problems, and depression. *Contemporary Family Therapy, 30,* 183–198.

Hargrave, T. D., & Pfitzer, P. F. (2003). *The new contextual therapy: Guiding the power of give and take.* New York, NY: Routledge.

Hatala, A. R. (2013). Towards a biopsychosocial-spiritual approach in health psychology: Exploring theoretical orientations and future directions. *Journal of Spirituality in Mental Health, 15,* 256–276.

Hibbs, B. J. (2009). *Try to see it my way: Being fair in love and marriage.* New York, NY: Penguin.

Hodgson, J., Lamson, A. L., & Reese, L. (2007). The biopsychosocial-spiritual interview method. *The therapist's notebook for family health care.* New York, NY: Haworth Press.

James, W. (1909). Confidences of a psychological researcher. *The American Magazine, 68,* p. 589.

McDaniel, S. M., Doherty, W. J., & Hepworth, J. (2014). *Medical family therapy and integrated care* (2nd ed.). Washington, DC: American Psychological Association.

Wright, L. M., Watson, W. L., & Bell, J. M. (1996) *Belief: The heart of healing in families and illness.* New York, NY: Basic Books.

Chapter 3

Capturing the Human Experience

The Role of Assessment

Although it would be impossible to find a foolproof way to explain the fullness of the human experience, the four dimensions found in the contextual approach provide a robust starting place to help clinicians begin connecting with and treating the patients and families with whom they work. We like to think of these contextual dimensions as an interactive map, like those found in much of today's technology. You can set a goal of where you'd like to start and end. For example, you can set a start point of Dallas and an end point of San Francisco, and the map provides you with an overview of what you'll need to know to get there. However, the technology also allows you to quickly and easily change your route to adjust to construction, traffic, scenic detours, and weather conditions.

We find the same to be true in clinical practice. We may have a multidimensional roadmap that guides us in a contextually focused assessment, but we can tailor that assessment to our clinical goals, our patients' needs and preferences, and the settings in which we work. We also recognize that clinicians' focus areas of the assessment will differ based upon their professional discipline, job description, and the amount of time they have to spend with patients and provide treatment. Therefore, we will strive to describe general aspects of assessment and intervention planning in this chapter so you can choose how to apply some of these principles within your practice of healthcare.

In this chapter, we will focus on how to effectively and efficiently gather assessment data using the four domains of contextual therapy, as augmented by the biopsychosocial-spiritual (BPSS model). We will provide some specific recommendations for clinical interview methods and examples of self-report measures targeting key contextual constructs. Finally, we will describe how to use those assessments to establish patient- and family-centered treatment goals, coordinate care across multiple providers, and evaluate progress over time.

ASSESSMENT: ALPHA BUT NOT OMEGA

Assessment is a good beginning to understanding how to help enact change, and the process should be always ongoing throughout the course of treatment. However, it is important to note that assessment is never an end in and of itself. In contextual therapy, assessment provides the clinician with "the ability to focus on the *causes* of behaviors and to view symptomology only in terms of *responses* to violations of love and trust" (Hargrave & Pfitzer, 2003, p. 41). Working within a contextual framework requires a focus on assessing and reassessing the thoughts, emotions, and behaviors of the individuals, couples, and families with whom you work.

Because this mode of therapy targets some of the most fundamental and sensitive topics of human relationships (such as trust and fairness), clinicians must develop a keen awareness of how to appropriately time and structure interventions. In order to do this well, you must first understand the factors contributing to why you're seeing this person (or persons) in the first place. A constant state of assessment, as opposed to giving it a finite place within the early stages of treatment, helps the clinician (1) learn what's important to the patient, (2) develop relevant, realistic goals for treatment, and (3) determine when it is appropriate to ask patients sensitive, probing, sometimes painful questions.

A thorough assessment should also be infused with strategies promoting multidirected partiality, the work that a clinician does to actively relate to and understand all individuals within the system. An analysis of Boszormenyi-Nagy's contextual therapy sessions revealed a simple way to infuse clinical work with multidirected partiality: organizing the structure of the session so that every family member gets a chance to speak about his or her point of view (van der Meiden, Noordegraaf, & van Ewijk, 2017). You must assess the perspectives of all who have some intersection with the problem at hand. In other words, a thorough assessment shouldn't be gathered through the eyes of just one person since multiple perspectives provide valuable lenses through which to view the problem (Cierpka, Thomas, & Sprenkle, 2005). Assessing the problem through multiple lenses and using the process of multidirected partiality to build rapport may help you realize during interventions when the process might need to slow down or take a different direction if engagement is dwindling for some within the system. Assessment of only one individual's perspective leaves room for blind spots.

In the current mental health system, treatment of patients is often driven by categorizing symptoms and delivering a diagnosis. Although assessment that leads to an individual diagnosis (depression, anxiety, etc.) can be useful at times for clinicians and patients, diagnosis and categorization must never be the end goal of treatment. For individual patients and their families, an overemphasis on diagnosis or a narrow-minded view of treatment options can be counterproductive, isolating, and stifling. The contextual framework includes an assessment of individual diagnoses but always within the context of relational symptoms that prohibit couples and families from functioning in fair and trustworthy ways. As Hargrave and Pfitzer (2003) concluded, diagnosis "is important for communication within the scientific community but offers only a few tools for treatment," which is why in contextual therapy, "the individual psychology dimension offers the psychotherapist an opportunity to view human beings outside of their symptomology" and assesses more than mental health symptoms (p. 41).

What to Ask

One of the most essential qualities for being a good researcher is being curious and knowing how to ask a good question. In a way, assessment can be considered a type of research. Instead of researching a particular topic, though, your job as a clinician is to be curious about the patient, explore the context surrounding the circumstances that brought the patient in to see you, and know how to ask questions that are likely to give you the information you need in order to make a good plan. A contextually focused biopsychosocial-spiritual assessment helps guide a clinician to ask questions about various dimensions of a patient's individual and family life. Assessment is also one way to build a relationship with a patient by showing respectful curiosity about what he or she has experienced.

This next section will include some questions we recommend asking and behavioral markers we recommend observing as part of a contextually focused biopsychosocial-spiritual assessment. Although we will use the four dimensions of the contextual framework to organize the assessment, we recognize that these dimensions often have considerable overlap, and questions from one dimension will often lead to follow-up questions more fitting for another dimension. This is similar to the inevitable interrelationships of constructs found in the biopsychosocial-spiritual (BPSS) approach. We consider these complex interactions to be a benefit of both the contextual framework and the BPSS approach. These recommendations are not all-inclusive, but they represent a starting place for learning to conceptualize patients' experience in a contextually focused, biopsychosocial-spiritual way. In preparation for the second section of this book, we will also focus on questions most likely to be relevant to families' experience of health and illness and how that intersects with relational health and well-being.

OBJECTIFIABLE FACTS

As you will recall from the previous chapter, objectifiable facts refer to factual circumstances such as life events and demographics. No matter what clinical setting you practice in, your intake form is likely to give you some background information about your patient. Common elements include name, age, race/ethnicity, gender, relationship status, home location, mental health history, and physical health history. Most often, these represent a snapshot of the patient's current situation. A thorough profile of past developments is often reserved for a clinical interview with a therapist, or perhaps more rarely, a more detailed form for evaluation purposes.

The biological component of the BPSS model reminds us to inquire for more details about health conditions, including past medical and mental health diagnoses, treatments used, and responses to treatments. One critical component of understanding the impact of health conditions includes the relationship between the timing of symptoms in the patient's life cycle stage and placement within the family life cycle (Carter & McGoldrick, 1989). In addition, current medical conditions should also be assessed, and clinicians should inquire about side effects of medication, time and energy involved in treatment regimens, and level of adherence to medical recommendations. It is also helpful to gather information about family history of illnesses, especially diseases with a known genetic component such as certain forms of breast cancer, type 1 diabetes, and Huntington's disease, or those with an environmental or lifestyle component such as asthma, human immunodeficiency virus (HIV), or type 2 diabetes. Similar information should be gathered about past and current mental health diagnoses. As healthcare costs in the United States expand, it would also be prudent to inquire about how patients pay for their medical services (e.g. private insurance or government-subsidized insurance such as Medicare or Medicaid) and whether they feel they have adequate funds to pay for healthcare. If ignored, facts like this leave a significant gap in creating a realistic treatment plan.

Medical providers are likely familiar with inquiring about family history of diseases, but the influence of family on health extends far beyond genetically and environmentally shared conditions. Families play an essential role in providing emotional and practical support during times of illness, so it is important to gather information about those who are blood relatives and those who are not but are still considered family. To get started, here are some sample questions:

- Who do you consider to be family? Is there anyone you're not related to by blood but consider to be in your closest circle of support? How nearby to you do these family members live, and how often are you in contact?

- Do you belong to a religious or spiritual group that provides you with support? How often do you engage in religious practices or spiritual experiences with others?

- What major losses has your family experienced during your lifetime? Were there any losses that occurred before you were born that influenced the way your family thinks about health and illness?

In this dimension, the clinician focuses on getting "just the facts," not inquiring about meanings attached to these events or illness experiences. The following dimensions build upon the foundation of the first dimension and encourage reflection about how these experiences have impacted individual functioning and social relationships.

INDIVIDUAL PSYCHOLOGY

Individual psychology includes individuals' internal motivation, perceptions, and reactions to the facts of life and our relationships with others. It has to do with how we make sense of our experiences and attach meaning to them, as well as personality characteristics and levels of self-esteem. This section can also include aspects of mental health diagnoses, such as those found in the Diagnostic and Statistical Manual V (DSM-V; American Psychiatric Association, 2013).

The role of mental health diagnoses is controversial. As Boszormenyi-Nagy and Krasner (1986) wrote, "At best, [diagnoses] have a somewhat predictive value in terms of a person's behavioral tendencies. At worst, diagnostic categories can be misleading" (p. 158). Two of the most convincing benefits of a system for naming mental health diagnoses relate to its ability to create a shared language between providers and to develop evidence-based treatments for a specified constellation of symptoms. Being able to name "what's going on" in terms of a commonly understood phenomenon (such as depression) can be relieving for individuals who recognize some kind of impairment or distress but are unsure of how to describe it or believe the myth that they experience problems due to some character flaw. There are, however, downsides to any system of categorization, including mental health diagnoses. Differences within groups (such as men with depression) are often grossly understated and poorly understood, some individuals blame decisions and behaviors on a diagnosis rather than accept personal responsibility, and diagnostic categories often fail to account for complexity and obscure unique aspects of individuals' lives that extend beyond a diagnosis. Using the process of multidirected partiality can help the clinician attend to various individuals' perspectives on the meanings and importance of diagnoses. Despite these challenges, mental health diagnoses are an important part of communicating with other healthcare professionals and receiving reimbursement from insurance companies, so we advocate for a cautious, thoughtful use of including mental health diagnoses as part of a thorough contextually focused BPSS assessment.

One way to build upon mental health diagnoses is to be intentional in remaining curious about unique aspects of individuals' thoughts, feelings, and behaviors. Never assume that a diagnosis or demographic variable explains all. One simple question we have used with patients to learn about their underlying motivations and value systems is to ask, "What are you passionate about in life?" Some patients, we have found, have a ready-made answer, and this often signals being a close connection to everyday life and one's value system. Answers to this question can be quite varied, including improving one's time in a competitive race, teaching in a low-income school district, or raising children to be responsible and polite. Many times, the answer to this question is related to a set of spiritual beliefs, sometimes encompassed within a set of religious practices. Some patients struggle to answer this question and will say, "I don't know what I'm passionate about. I feel like I lost sight of that years ago," which often signals to us that we need to tap into more of what the patient previously found valuable and inspiring in their work, hobbies, and personal relationships.

Why ask this question, "What are you passionate about in life?" This question is fundamental as to how people make decisions about how they spend money and time, how they interact with others, whom they spend time with, and what drives them to work through difficulties and struggles. Our opinion is that a core part of individual psychology concerns value systems and passions: key driving forces in decision-making. To help patients make thoughtful, informed decisions about how to remain healthy and work toward healing in the context of healing, we must know what fuels their efforts or stalls them from making progress.

As we mentioned in the previous chapter, individual psychology can also include how individuals make sense out of experiences that promote love, trust, and loyalty with others. At times, we all get caught up in cognitive distortions such as catastrophizing a negative experience, assigning blame to ourselves that doesn't belong to us, or getting stuck in tunnel vision with a narrow view. Throughout the next few chapters, we will provide some examples of how experiences that promote or detract from a balanced relational ethic influence the ways in which individuals attach meaning to their relationships with themselves and others, as well as emotional states and repetitive thought processes.

SYSTEMIC INTERACTIONS

Although knowing about an individual's experiences in life and how they make sense of them is important, it does not provide a complete assessment. Retaining an individualized focus will only get us so far in conceptualizing the underlying issues inhibiting the health and functioning of the patients whom we serve. As systemic thinkers, we know the importance of understanding how individuals are influenced by and influence their environmental and relational context. Assessing this third dimension of systemic interactions provides a deeper understanding of how individuals interact with their families when making decisions, how their beliefs and health behaviors are similar to or different from those of their families of origin, and what patterns of communication and behavior they use in order to seek support from loved ones during times of difficulty. Although there are many different factors that contribute to family health, from a contextual perspective a patient's "capacity to problem solve, to change according to the family life cycle, to balance closeness and distance, to respect boundaries between the generations, and to develop and maintain a common belief system" are of upmost importance (Hargrave & Pfitzer, 2003, p. 51).

When you use a contextual perspective to guide your clinical work, you remain intentional in recognizing the importance of all your patient's relationships and are curious about how those relationships impact the patient's day-to-day functioning and overall meaning taken from their experiences. You inquire about how other family members would react to certain decisions or actions, and you work diligently to give credit to worthwhile efforts that contribute to trust, fairness, and mutual caring. This happens regardless of how many people are in the room with you, meaning that you consider familial context even if they're not present in the exam room or counseling room that day. Regarding systemic interactions, we consider the "power, competition, coalitions, and alliances" of family members and how these relationships dynamics are contributing to the overall health of the patients and their families (Heusden & Eerenbeemt, 1987, p. 97).

One way to better understand complex, fast-moving family dynamics is by taking time to reflect on how you notice families communicate with each other (when you're fortunate enough to have them in the same room as each other) or communicate about each other (when they talk individually about each other to you). Communication provides the pathway for "members [to] know how they are regarded and what rules and beliefs govern their interactions" (Hargrave & Pfitzer, 2003, p. 47). As we continually assess communication patterns, we take note of the amounts of empathy, patience, accommodation, and forgiveness that already exist within each relationship, and we look for opportunities to overtly call that into recognition and offer credit for communication styles that promote trustworthiness and care. Likewise, we also look for the presence of contempt, harsh criticism, defensiveness, disengagement, and other communicational patterns that threaten emotional safety and trust within relationships (Gottman, 1994). As Watzlawick, Bavelas, and Jackson (2011) wrote, "No matter how one may try, one cannot not communicate. Activity or inactivity, words or silence all have message value" and convey some meaning to others (p 30). Thus, an assessment of communication should include verbal content as well as silent pauses, nonverbal gestures and facial expressions, the timing of responses and how they relate to others' responses, types of imagery evoked, and much more. What makes the contextual analysis of communication unique is how the clinician looks for the ways in which these communication strategies are related to expressions of trust, loyalty, and fairness.

This dimension represents one way in which the contextual framework and the biopsychosocial-spiritual approach are intertwined yet focus on separate pieces of a similar construct: social context and relationships. The contextual dimension of systemic interactions builds upon the BPSS approach of recognizing the importance of social relationships to gather an in-depth assessment of how exactly those relationships impact psychological, spiritual, relational, and biomedical health and gives specific guidance on concepts to assess (e.g. power, alliances between certain members, coalitions against other members). Similarly, the final contextual dimension of relational ethics adds additional understanding to the ways in which our factual experiences, beliefs and motivations, and relationship dynamics influence our perception of trustworthiness and fairness. These concepts are essential for individual health and well-being across the biopsychosocial spectrum.

RELATIONAL ETHICS

How couples and families interact with each other in the present moment is inextricably linked to memories of past interactions and the meanings attached to those experiences. Likewise, the ways in which we interact with those around us sets in motion a series of events and ways of thinking and being that influence future generations who are affected by the consequences of our choices today, both positive and negative. As we have previously mentioned, the cornerstone construct of contextual therapy is relational ethics (Boszormenyi-Nagy & Krasner, 1986). As Hargrave and Pfitzer (2003) explained, "Our work, actions, emotions, contributions, distractions, and destructiveness all become part of the legacy, heritage and foundation that we pass along to others. These 'others' may be part of our biological family relationships or may be part of the people we have made family by our commitments and love" (p. 71).

An important note to start: assessment of relational ethics does not require judgment. The job of a contextual clinician is not to act as judge and jury to determine how ethical relationships are. Rather, the clinician's job is to help individuals and families assess their own relationships to determine areas where balance and justice exist, as well as areas that require change to improve the ethical nature of this relationship. In the most basic sense, we look for ways in which relationships have become unbalanced or overburdened for one person or another. We look for signs that point us to the presence or absence of trustworthiness, loyalty, and a commitment to justice within the couple or family system.

The expectations that people have of themselves and others in their relationships are highlighted through relational ethics (Hargrave & Pfitzer, 2003). Relational ethics addresses the balance of what people feel obligated to give in their relationships and what they feel entitled to receive in their relationships. Notice that this isn't limited to tangible things like, "I expect us to spend Christmas at home with my family if we spend Thanksgiving with yours." These expectations, spoken or unspoken, also include ideas like, "I expect us to stay together even if one of us is diagnosed with a terminal illness that requires a lot of caregiving, and I want you to let me take care of you at home" or "I feel loved when you take time to listen to my complaints about my physical pain instead of just dismissing me." Thus, an important part of assessing relational ethics includes understanding the expectations that each member has about how to give and receive love, care, trustworthiness, and loyalty, especially in contexts of illness and uncertainty. Uncovering the balance of relational ethics can be as simple as asking about how family members show care for one another (van der Meiden et al., 2017).

This dimension of contextual therapy can also be known as the power of giving-and-receiving in relationships. As individual members balance the giving-and-receiving in their relationship and assume responsibility for their actions, trustworthiness can be increased (Hargrave, Jennings, & Anderson, 1991), and the relationship becomes more stable. An unfairly balanced relationship is not one that meets all members' needs and has the flexibility to withstand changes over time. A clinician working from a contextual framework intentionally seeks to understand how individuals show and receive love, trust, and loyalty within the relationship. Entitlements can also include a need for respect, care, and intimacy within relationships (Hargrave & Pfitzer, 2003). In fitting with the human desire for justice and fairness, these concepts should be balanced *over time* between who gives and receives this type of care, and that contributes to an overall healthy relationship that supports all members.

This balance in relationships is often thought of as a relational ledger. This ledger includes one column for what you give to the relationship, and one column for what you receive from the relationship. Ideally, these two columns would stabilize in length over time, even though they may look different at various stages throughout the course of a relationship. As clinicians, we have found a simple, useful exercise for individuals or family members who are expressing a sense of unfairness or imbalance in their relationship is to draw out a ledger to differentiate between what they perceive themselves as giving to and receiving from those within their partnership or family. Since imbalance can be such a difficult, intense concept to clearly identify and talk about, this method (1) slows down the conversation when resentment or anger is inhibiting progress and (2) begins a dialogue about what a fairer balance that is acceptable to all might look like.

After reaching a certain threshold of violations of love, trust, and loyalty, some people reach a tipping point and act in ways that are destructive to others (and ultimately themselves, too). For instance, a father might feel justified in exploding into angry, belittling, and demeaning outbursts toward his children since this was the same treatment that he received from his parents. He feels he knows no other way. Due to the past hurts the father has received in his life and the toll that takes on his current well-being, he might even become blind to seeing how his actions are impacting others. This unbalance of burdens in the father's life can be felt throughout multiple generations of the family system, and it will certainly affect his children's relationship with him and how they carry those expectations forward into relationships with others. What could a contextually minded clinician do in this type of situation? The clinician's job is to help each member of a system feel validated and honor the ways in which each person has been hurt by an injustice, working to increase the empathy and understanding of other family members and their perspectives. Van der Meiden et al. (2017) wrote, "Instead of attacking the [parent] for this injurious behavior toward the child, the most effective intervention is to show partiality toward his or her own past childhood victimization" (p. 8). Then, restorative work to bring a new balance of trust and fairness for the current generation (and future ones) can begin.

As you help patients and their families rebalance and mend painful relationships, you must also be mindful in acknowledging the powerful role that loyalty plays in families. As Boszormenyi-Nagy and Krasner (1986) explained, "loyalty is the glue of parent-child relationships" (p. 145). Loyalty helps bind family members together and keeps them committed to one another, even in the most challenging circumstances where trust and fairness are questioned. Assessing for loyalty in relational ethics requires an awareness of topics such as grief and loss, family secrets, and myths (Hargrave & Pfitzer, 2003). As explained by Hargrave and Pfitzer (2003), "Loyalty is powerful in relationships because it essentially proclaims our priority and thereby suggests an organization or hierarchy of how we will go about meeting obligations and receiving entitlements" (p. 80). Since family relationships are the very first relationships that we experience, we are compelled to put them first even if this may require great sacrifice (Hargrave & Pfitzer, 2003). This loyalty to family can sometime create conflict within relationships. For instance, a husband may wonder why his wife feels such a strong need to visit her parents or attend family gatherings rather than attend social events with his friends, and this may lead to the husband's perception of the relationship as unfairly sided with his wife's family of origin. Similarly, the wife may feel caught in a loyalty conflict when making decisions about whether to prioritize the need of her family of origin or her husband.

For clinicians who are experienced working within a contextual framework and for those who are new to the model, it can be difficult to ask about the abstract concepts found in the relational ethics dimension. To help you get started, here are some questions that you may consider asking in order to better understand your clients' experiences of trust, loyalty, and fairness. Depending upon therapeutic goals and the phase of therapeutic interventions, various types of questions can serve different purposes.

For example, these questions can lead to opportunities to show empathy and provide an opportunity to give credit for the past hurts patients have experienced in their relationships. Although they're grouped by main idea, we recommend starting with one question from a group at a time and working your way through the questions slowly and as applicable to patients' responses.

- In the relationships with your family of origin (parents, siblings, grandparents, etc.) have you experienced any violations of love, trust, or loyalty? In other words, has it been difficult to trust any of your family members or their loyalty to you and your relationship? Are there family members who should have been more empathetic and loving toward you, but were not?

- When you think about the relationships you have with your family members, do any of these relationships feel unfair or unbalanced? For instance, have you felt that you contribute much more to one of these relationships than you receive in return? How long has this relationship felt unfair, and when did it begin to feel this way? What are your expectations of what you should give in these relationships? What do you believe you are entitled to receive in return?

- Have there been times in which you've had to make difficult choices to prioritize the needs of one person you care about over the needs of another person you love? How did you decide whose needs took priority? Does this seem to be pretty standard, or was that out of the ordinary for you to set the priorities in this way? How has this affected your relationship with both of these people?

This second set of questions can help clinicians acknowledge the efforts of their patients to sustain their relationships and the contributions they have made to a more positive, healing environment. It is important to note that although we use the word "family," a reference to neighborhood, community, or close friends could also be appropriate.

- In what ways do you believe that you have tried to contribute to your family relationships? How have your efforts contributed to the success of your relationships and had a positive impact?
- Are there ways that you have sacrificed for other family members or put their needs above your own? Have your family members acknowledged the efforts you are making in these relationships? How have they shown their appreciation for your sacrifices?
- In what way have your family members contributed to the success of your relationships with them? How do you show them gratitude? How well do they receive your gratitude?

A Contextually Focused Genogram

Including a genogram in clinical assessment can be a valuable tool as you begin formulating your conceptualization of changes needed to restore health and functioning. The genogram provides a visual framework for mapping family patterns and has been used by clinicians for over 50 years to assess and understand relationships (McGoldrick, 2012). There are two ways of thinking about how genograms intersect with the building of a therapeutic relationship. On the one hand, an established, trusting therapeutic relationship can help the patient feel more comfortable in sharing sensitive information about family relationships and historical experiences. On the other hand, sharing stories can be a way to build vulnerability and earn trust in a new therapist if the concept is introduced in a respectful, curious way with appropriate timing and reasoning.

The genogram is a similar tool to a nursing or genetics pedigree, but its main purpose is to represent patterns of relational behavior within the family structure rather than track the presence or absence of health conditions. A genogram includes multiple types of family information, such as "who is in the family, the dates of their births, marriages, moves, illnesses, deaths, primary characteristics and level of functioning of different family members, education, occupation, psychological and physical health, successes and failures . . . closeness, conflict, or cut off" (McGoldrick, 2012, p. 1).

Employing a genogram in your work with patients can be an illuminating experience because it allows you to examine the family from multiple perspectives and understand patterns and descriptions of relationships (McGoldrick, 2012). Using a genogram to understand ways in which family members perceive the relationships they have with each other can be a useful predeterminant to using the intervention of multidirected partiality to demonstrate active empathy for multiple perspectives within the family (Sibley et al., 2016). A contextually focused genogram can allow you to map out how individuals perceive the balance of fairness within relationships and to explore the violations of love, trust, and loyalty in both horizontal and vertical relationships. Using a basic framework of genograms as described by McGoldrick (2012), combined with additional contextual elements of fairness, love, trust, loyalty, and entitlements in relationships, creates a more comprehensive, multidimensional picture of the functioning of families over multiple generations. In this way, clinicians and patients can visually make sense of patterns of unfairness and unethical relational behavior that may be impeding patient and family functioning. Insight into these patterns may help make sense of multidimensional factors that contribute to psychological and emotional distress, often manifested in physical symptoms and detrimental health behaviors. We believe that co-creating this contextually focused genogram with patients has the potential to lead to an increase of insight and meaning-making for both the patients and their family members.

Consider this story. When Cameron was 15 years old, his father Paul was diagnosed with Parkinson's disease. This chronic illness presented enormous challenges that complicated family life and strained relationships that had already been tested. Although this disease took its toll on everyone in the family, Cameron felt that he was unduly affected by his father's disease. For as long as he could remember, Cameron had felt as if he did not receive as much attention from his father as his siblings received. As the youngest child, he was often forgotten by the other members of his family who were attending to the physical and emotional needs of his father and taking care of their own business. For instance, although Paul attended Darin and Jared's football games and Haley's piano recitals, he often said he was too tired to go and watch Cameron's baseball games and seemed uninterested when Cameron talked to him about baseball. Generally, only Cameron's mother Allison was present at his baseball games. Throughout Cameron's childhood and adolescence, he consistently felt that his relationship with his father was unfair. Over time, he learned not to trust his father after years of seeking Paul's acceptance and love.

Now an adult, Cameron has been unable to repair the relationship with his father, and it is not uncommon for the two to spend six months not speaking to one another. In his early twenties, Cameron made the decision to emotionally distance himself from the other men in his family, as well, since he felt they would see him in a negative light if they knew about the distance between him and his father. When he is with these other men, he often acts cold, argumentative, and selfish in his interactions with them. As a protective defense mechanism, Cameron had developed a reliance on destructive entitlement, focusing on himself. This made it challenging for him to accept or understand any of their perspectives on family life since Cameron could only think of himself and the hurt he had experienced.

After living with Parkinson's disease for the past 20 years, Paul's health has substantially begun to deteriorate, and his physicians believe he only has a few months to live. In these few short months that Paul has left to live, Cameron must decide what type of relationship he will have with his father before he dies. Paul's long-standing depression symptoms have worsened, and his primary care physician refers him and his family to seek counseling to grieve and process how to repair family relationships during the short time he has left to live. As the therapist treating Paul's family, the genogram you create might look something like Figure 3.1.

USING GENOGRAMS WITHIN THE MEDICAL SETTING

Traditionally, genograms have been used most often in outpatient mental health settings by trained counselors and therapists. Although there are certainly variations across clients and therapists, a thorough

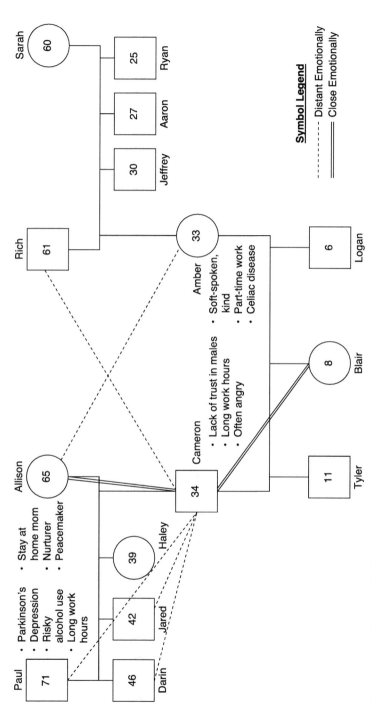

Figure 3.1 *A Contextually Focused Genogram*

genogram of multiple generations can take one to two 50-minute therapy sessions to complete. The therapist and client(s) may complete the genogram together as the therapist learns about the client's background, and it may be revised over time as nuances of relationships are revealed and changes occur. In more long-term therapy experiences with an intensive focus on family relationships and its impact on functioning, this is certainly appropriate.

However, therapists who work in more time-limited settings do not have the luxury of spending several valuable therapy hours to complete a rigorous genogram with detailed descriptions of relationships between all members. This is certainly the case for therapists who work with patients and their families using brief interventions or a very limited number of focused therapy sessions in medical settings such as primary care clinics, specialty care clinics, or limited hospital stays. These therapists must creatively find ways to adapt the use of genograms to gather relevant, sensitive information in a short time span and apply that to planned interventions in order to reduce symptoms and restore functioning.

To effectively and efficiently use genograms in time-limited medical settings, we provide several recommendations for mental health clinicians and non-therapist providers:

- Providing some context for why you might be asking questions about historical family relationships is helpful for patients who have never had a genogram completed before.

- Complete the genogram in a transparent way with patients (and their families, if applicable)—that is, with them in the room as opposed to following a visit with them. Determine how you will store this living document in your electronic health record and document changes over time.

- Don't worry about having a perfect genogram as you sketch it out. It will be messy and change over time as you get more information. It takes time to put all the pieces together.

- Identify the core people in the patient's support system, and ask about how they play a role in the current presenting problem(s) and how they impact the functioning of various family members.

- To add contextual elements to the genogram, you can ask questions like, "When you were sick with _____, who did you find to be the most trustworthy person to provide you with care? How balanced do you feel the relationship is between you and your other siblings in helping to care for your parents as they get older? Are there any people in your family you feel torn between as you make decisions about how to balance your time? As you work on better managing _____, who do you think will be your most loyal supporter?" Any ways in which you can connect these types of questions to care plans and established goals for patients will be most beneficial.

Structured Assessments: Futile or Useful?

Within the field of couple and family therapy, there is a long history of lively debate concerning the utility and appropriateness of structured, validated clinical assessments. Although Sherman and Fredman (1987, p 5) cheekily wrote, "That which can be measured may be irrelevant," the value of structured assessments comes from their ability to gather data in an objective manner, compare individuals' responses with national norms, and help identify areas of concern. However, there are also downsides, which include time intensiveness and expenses of some tests and a lack of connection with an underlying model of clinical intervention (Gehart, 2010).

Although there may not be a strong consensus within the field of psychotherapy, the same dissent is not generally shared within the medical community. The current model of western medicine is built upon formal assessments guiding plans for treatment. These assessments are also essential for receiving payment for services rendered through commercial insurers and government-subsidized insurance programs. Practice transformation efforts to create models of advanced primary care eligible for value-based payments are tied to assessing and demon-strating measurable outcomes with improved health outcomes and decreased financial costs (Hudak & Shenkin, 2016). Thus, therapists who work within a medical clinic or collaborate closely with physicians and other healthcare professionals do not have the luxury of choosing whether to conduct formal assessments; quantitative assessment data is a prerequisite for effective communication and documentation within these settings. These therapists are faced with the challenge of determining what role structured assessments hold within their clinical practice and how they will use information gathered to plan and conduct treatment in a way meaningful to them, their patients, and other professionals involved in their patients' care.

There is a myriad of commonly used structured assessments to screen for individual diagnoses such as depression, anxiety, attention deficit hyperactivity disorder, bipolar disorder, and dementia. These are commonly found in primary care and other medical settings, and we advocate the use of these instruments when appropriate for the setting and for the benefit of the patient. Likewise, the couple and family therapy field has produced several well-validated measurements to assess relational functioning, and a significant number of them are described by Sherman and Fredman (1987). In this section, we present two structured assessments that are grounded in the contextual therapy framework: the Relational Ethics Scale (RES) and the Fairness Questionnaire. For clinicians wishing to create a starting point for discussion contextual topics with patients, we recommend these scales as excellent beginnings.

RELATIONAL ETHICS SCALE

Perhaps the most well-known, research-supported scale that specifically assesses contextual constructs such as trustworthiness and justice, loyalty, and entitlement to receive care is the Relational Ethics Scale (RES; Hargrave, Jennings, & Anderson, 1991). The RES is a 24-item scale designed to measure contextual therapy's construct of relational ethics; the sense of justice and fairness within families. The RES asks subjects to respond to questions using a five-item Likert scale format, ranging from one (*strongly disagree*) to five (*strongly agree*). Twelve items are reverse-coded, and higher scores indicate higher levels of relational ethics (i.e. more trust and fairness, more loyalty, and less destructive entitlement). The instrument has been normed with adults from a variety of socioeconomic, racial, and marital status backgrounds (Hargrave et al., 1991; Hargrave & Bomba, 1993).

The RES includes eight subscales (vertical trust and justice, vertical loyalty, vertical entitlement, horizontal trust and justice, horizontal loyalty, horizontal entitlement, total vertical relational ethics, and total horizontal relational ethics). As you will recall from previous chapters, vertical relationships are those hierarchical connections between parents and children, and horizontal relationships are those non-hierarchical connections between siblings and romantic partners. In contextual therapy, trust and justice provide the foundation for all other relational ethics constructs and are evidenced by an overall balance of giving and taking in relationships (Hargrave et al., 1991). An example of a question measuring trust and justice is "This person listens to me and values my thoughts." Loyalty can be defined as a sense of commitment to the relationship based upon merit earned by nature of being part of that relationship (Boszormenyi-Nagy & Krasner, 1986), and a sample question is "I try to meet the emotional needs of this person." Entitlement in the RES measures how individuals perceive whether they have received what they deserve from their family members and partners (Hargrave et al., 1991), with higher scores indicating a stronger belief that the individual received what he or she was due. An example of a question measuring entitlement is "When I feel angry, I tend to take it out on this person."

How might you use the Relational Ethics Scale in your clinical practice? This instrument presents an excellent opportunity to learn more about experiences within patients' families of origin and their current relationships with a romantic partner. We recognize that this scale is unlikely to be relevant for all patients seeking treatment for health issues, so we recommend the use of this scale with patients experiencing some or all of the following:

- Difficulty making medical decisions or adhering to treatment recommendations due to loyalty conflicts within the family (feeling pulled between obligations to multiple people)
- Rigid beliefs about who should or should not be involved in the caregiving process for themselves or other family members who are ill
- Trouble engaging desired levels of support from family members or friends during health problems
- Unclear or narrow-sighted expectations of others and what support they should provide during illness
- Difficulty establishing a trusting relationship with the treatment team when familial difficulties are also known to be part of the patient's history.

The questions contained in the RES are likely to target constructs such as problems with trustworthiness, loyalty, and balanced giving and taking that influenced patients' engagement with the healthcare system and their beliefs about illness and caregiving. The RES can be administered in a relatively short amount of time, with most people being able to complete the measure within 7–10 minutes. When time is short, however, the clinician could consider using just a few selected questions from the scale in her conversation with the family as a topic of discussion to learn more about how experiences within the patient's family of origin and couple relationships have influenced expectations about health and illness (see Table 3.1).

Table 3.1   Relational Ethics Scale

1 Strongly agree	2 Agree	3 Neutral	4 Disagree	5 Strongly disagree

Vertical Relational Ethics

1. I could trust my family to seek my best interests.	1	2	3	4	5
2. Individuals that were in my family were blamed for problems that were not their fault.*	1	2	3	4	5
3. Pleasing one of my parents often meant displeasing the other.*	1	2	3	4	5
4. I received the love and affection from my family that I deserved.	1	2	3	4	5
5. No matter what happened, I always stood by my family.	1	2	3	4	5
6. At times, it seemed that one or both of my parents disliked me.*	1	2	3	4	5
7. Love and warmth were given equally to all family members.	1	2	3	4	5
8. At times, I was used by my family unfairly.*	1	2	3	4	5
9. I felt my life was dominated by my parents' desires.*	1	2	3	4	5
10. Individuals in my family were willing to give of themselves to benefit the family.	1	2	3	4	5
11. I continue to seek closer relationships with my family.	1	2	3	4	5
12. I often feel deserted by my family.*	1	2	3	4	5

Horizontal Relational Ethics

13. I try to meet the emotional needs of this person.	1	2	3	4	5
14. I do not trust this individual to look out for my best interests.*	1	2	3	4	5
15. When I feel hurt, I say or do hurtful things to this person.*	1	2	3	4	5
16. This person stands beside me in times of trouble or joy.	1	2	3	4	5

17. Before I make important decisions, I ask for the opinion of this person.	1	2	3	4	5
18. There is unequal contribution to the relationship between me and this individual.*	1	2	3	4	5
19. When I feel angry, I tend to take it out on this person.*	1	2	3	4	5
20. We are equal partners in this relationship.	1	2	3	4	5
21. We give of ourselves to benefit one another.	1	2	3	4	5
22. I take advantage of this individual.*	1	2	3	4	5
23. I am taken for granted or used unfairly in this relationship.*	1	2	3	4	5
24. This person listens to me and values my thoughts.	1	2	3	4	5

Notes
* Item is reverse scored. Reprinted with permission from Hargrave et al (1991).

Fairness Questionnaire

Other well-known contextual writers, Hibbs and Getzen (2009), developed a Fairness Questionnaire that can be used to explore contextual topics with patients in a conversation-friendly way. One major difference between the RES and the Fairness Questionnaire is that the latter does not have empirical research validating its use as a clinical measure. However, the Fairness Questionnaire is still a useful tool to identify patterns pertaining to giving and taking, which may be immensely helpful to families struggling to define what seems fair in caring for sick members. The scoring for the Fairness Questionnaire is much simpler since responses are either "usually true" or "usually false." A few sample questions include:

- I go out on a limb for other people but am disappointed that they rarely do the same for me.
- I find myself excusing other people's behavior most of the time and then unexpectedly blowing up at small things.
- I want my spouse to automatically know what I need.
- When faced with the thought of discussing a problem with my partner, I decide "it's not worth it" because little or nothing will really change.
- I feel caught between my spouse and my parents on a regular basis.
- I feel disappointed in my kids much of the time for their insensitivity toward me.

A complete list of questions from the questionnaire can be found in Hibbs and Getzen (2009), and there are sections specific to fairness in relationships with partners, parents, and children. The patient-friendly, easy-to-understand language in the questionnaire can help illuminate if patients feel they are giving too much or too little in their relationships and how that impacts the support they give and receive during times of illness.

Assessment for Effective, Focused Intervention

There is an inextricable relationship between conducting assessment and crafting interventions. Once we better understand where breakdowns in relational ethics have occurred and how they influence individual and family functioning, we can create tailored interventions to help families create a legacy of health and take actions toward restoring trustworthiness, fairness, and loyalty. Crafting interventions without paying close attention to how we are assessing our patients and their families is akin to beginning to build a house without any blueprint and procurement of supplies. It just does not create a product that lasts.

What are the risks associated with a shoddy assessment that is too narrow, too vague and broad, or too single-sided? We fail to give ourselves enough information to truly know, to intimately understand, and to act in an informed way to help those who seek our care. When we do not take the time to really get to know our patients within their individual *and* relational contexts, we deprive ourselves of the opportunity to learn about their world—past, present, and future—and how it collides with our own. We too quickly make assumptions about what change our patients desire and what they need from us to seek that change. Perhaps most importantly, we communicate the faulty, naïve message that change can occur without understanding the roots of why change is needed and what might get in the way.

If you are sitting with an uncomfortable feeling that assessment is an important responsibility and a lengthy process, you're right. The job is never really finished. And as much as that can sound like a burden, it also is ripe with many opportunities for growing and learning and connecting. A good assessment saves time in the long run and creates more efficient, effective interventions. Fortunately, today's healthcare system is trending toward comprehensive, holistic care that attends to patients' bodies, minds, and spirits. The verdict is in: the only way to do this well is to work within a team of providers who have expertise across and within these domains. Comprehensive, holistic healthcare isn't just the job of the medical provider, nor the behavioral health providers with whom they work. Rather, assessing and understanding how to craft solid interventions is a responsibility that rests on the shoulders of all members of a patient's care team. Fortunately, for non-therapist clinicians who haven't previously been trained in contextual concepts but want to learn more about how to implement them into caring for patients and their families, there are always opportunities to seek support from therapists who have had training in contextual therapy.

REFERENCES

American Psychiatric Association (2013). Diagnosis and statistical manual of the mental disorders (5th ed.). Washington, DC: Author.

Boszormenyi-Nagy, I. & Krasner, B. R. (1986). *Between give and take: A clinical guide to contextual therapy.* New York, NY: Brunner/Mazel.

Carter, E. A. & McGoldrick, M. (1989). *The changing family life cycle: A framework for family therapy.* Boston: Allyn and Bacon.

Cierpka, M., Thomas, V., & Sprenkle, D. (2005). *Family assessment: Integrating multiple clinical perspectives.* Cambridge, MA: Hogrefe & Huber.

Gehart, D. (2010). Clinical assessment (pp. 53–86). In *Mastering competencies in family therapy: A practical approach to theories and clinical case documentation.* Belmont, CA: Brooks/Cole.

Gottman, J. (1994). *Why marriages succeed or fail . . . and how you can make yours last.* New York, NY: Fireside.

Hargrave, T. D., Jennings, G., & Anderson, W. (1991). The development of a relational ethics scale. *Journal of Marital and Family Therapy, 17*(2), 145–158.

Hargrave, T. D. & Bomba, A. K. (1993). Further validation of the relational ethics scale. *Journal of Marital and Family Therapy, 19*(3), 292–299.

Hargrave, T. D. & Pfitzer, P. F. (2003). *The new contextual therapy: Guiding the power of give and take.* New York, NY: Routledge.

Heusden, A. & Eerenbeemt, E. M. (1987). *Balance in motion: Ivan Boszormenyi-Nagy and his vision of individual and family therapy.* New York: Brunner/Mazel.

Hibbs, B. J. & Getzen, K. J. (2009). *Try to see it my way: Being fair in love and marriage.* New York: Avery.

Hudak, M. L. & Shenkin, B. N. (2016, March 18). Practice transformation: Quest for 'triple aim' fuels changes in payment methodology. Retrieved February 25, 2018 from www.aappublications.org/news/2016/03/18/PracticeTransformation031816

McGoldrick, M. (2012). *The genogram format for mapping family systems.* Retrieved February 25, 2018 from http://multiculturalfamily.org/publications/genogram-life-stories/

Sherman, R., & Fredman, N. (1987). Introduction to marriage and family testing (pp. 3–16). In *Handbook of measurements for marriage and family therapy.* Philadelphia, PA: Brunner/Mazel.

Sibley, D. S., Schmidt, A. E., & Kimmes, J. G. (2016). Applying a contextual therapy framework to treat panic disorder. A case study. *Journal of Family Psychotherapy, 24*(4), 299–317.

van der Meiden, J., Noordegraf, M., & van Ewjik, H. (2017). Applying the paradigm of relational ethics into contextual therapy. Analyzing the practice of Boszormenyi-Nagy. *Journal of Marital and Family Therapy.* doi: 10.1111/jmft.12262

Watzlawick, P., Bavelas, J. B., & Jackson, D. (2011). Pragmatics of human communication: A study of interactional patterns, pathologies, and paradoxes. New York, NY: Norton.

Chapter 4

Contextual Supervision
Helping Clinicians Find Balance

If you are a trained mental health professional reading this book, you are familiar with the concept of supervision. If you are not a mental health professional, you may be wondering, "What does supervision mean in this context?" Todd and Storm (2014) defined supervision as a relationship where one professional (a supervisee) seeks guidance from another professional (a supervisor) in order to advance the supervisee's clinical and professional competencies and ensure the provision of high-quality services for clients. Professional counselors, couple and family therapists, psychologists, and social workers are generally required to engage in clinical supervision in order to develop clinical skills in helping enact therapeutic change, manage administrative tasks, and process how their work intersects with their personal beliefs and values.

The core tenets of contextual supervision presented in this chapter will be most familiar to those trained in a mental health discipline. However, we will also make a case for including key contextual constructs in the training of non-mental health professionals who provide direct patient care at various points along the biopsychosocial continuum. The first part of this chapter will describe the "nuts and bolts" of contextual supervision for therapists, and the second part will address broader applications of contextual supervision constructs in the family-centered education of medically oriented providers and staff in healthcare.

PART I: CONTEXTUAL SUPERVISION FOR THERAPISTS

What is Unique About Contextual Supervision?

In the marriage and family therapy supervision literature, authors have primarily written about the modern and post-modern approaches of supervision. Despite being considered a modern theory, not much has been written about the contextual approach to supervision. This is unfortunate because contextual supervision offers supervisees the opportunity for additional insights to their clinical cases that other theories of supervision may overlook. Regarding contextual supervision, Roberto (2002) wrote:

> In families that do not show trustworthiness, merit, consideration for each other's efforts, or acknowledgment of loyalty, there are enormous consequences such as lack of self-awareness, behavioral symptoms and missing empathy. Contextual supervision focuses on teasing out the status of these "relational ethics" in client families by aiding the therapist to weigh the fairness, mutuality, and balance of family interactions with clients (p. 163).

The clear focus on fairness within family relationships is one way that contextual supervision is unique and it sets it apart when compared to other systemic forms of clinical supervision. Contextual supervision, however, includes far more than simply encouraging supervisees to focus on fairness. In one way or another, all of the contextual therapy principles and concepts contained in our previous chapters can be applied to work with supervisees in supervision, just as they can be applied to work with clients in therapy. The steps of multidirected partiality (empathy, crediting of both constructive and destructive elements of relationships, acknowledgment of efforts, and accountability) can each be used as a framework to guide clinical supervision case consultations and interactions with each supervisee. Sude and Gambrel (2017) even proposed that the same elements of trustworthiness, reciprocal giving and receiving, and fairness found in intergenerational family relationships can be applied to training and supervisory relationships as the trainer and trainee take turns teaching and learning from one another.

One of the most important benefits of using a contextual framework in supervision is that it does not require use in isolation. This means that the supervisee does not need to use contextual therapy as his primary model of therapy, nor does the supervisee need to operate solely from a contextual frame of reference. Rather, underlying tenets of contextual therapy and supervision can be used strategically to supplement other theoretical orientations a supervisor may use to guide his or her work and expand case conceptualization with supervisees.

Contextual Supervision Focus Areas

One of the primary functions of contextual supervision is to assist supervisees in recognizing the multiple perspectives of individuals in family systems by taking a stance of multidirected partiality. The supervisor encourages each supervisee to be accountable for acknowledging the viewpoints of all those who are involved in resolving a problem. In this way, supervisors can help promote balance and fairness within the relationships of the individuals, couples, and families with whom the supervisee may be working.

As explained by Brooks and Roberto-Forman (2014), contextual supervision specifically "focuses on teasing out these relational ethics by aiding supervisees to look for generational entitlement issues, fairness, mutuality, and balance in family interactions. Instead of being neutral, contextual therapists seek to be a resource of concern and support" in identifying areas of strained relational ethics (p. 196). Contextual supervision is an active approach of engaging supervisees in a way that will empathetically challenge their supervisees to consider alternative ways to address issues in therapy, bravely and compassionately address injustices that have occurred in clients' lives, and recognize client perspectives that they may not have previously considered. Just as contextual therapists would use the intervention of multidirected partiality with clients, contextual supervisors employ multidirected partiality with their supervisees to assess whether the supervisee understands and recognizes the various perspectives of the family members with whom they are working, as well as key stakeholders involved in the case (e.g. referring physician, case manager, teachers at school, etc.). Although there are many ways to approach contextual concepts, we have provided below a sampling of key issues likely to be addressed in contextual supervision.

Identifying Fairness Issues

One of the most worthwhile aspects of supervision approached from any theoretical lens is that it provides a therapist with the space to conceptualize clinical cases with a seasoned clinician who can bring additional insights into the issues that individuals, couples, and families are experiencing. In contextual therapy, this unique insight often centers around the ways in which fairness issues are infused within the problems clients bring to therapy. Consistent with the contextual therapy tradition, the supervisor makes sure that every family member's perspective is acknowledged, and that the clinician is actively considering even those outside of therapy who will be impacted by the decisions made during therapy. Some questions supervisors may use to address fairness issues could be:

- What do you believe are some of the most prominent fairness issues that your clients are experiencing in their relationships?

- How have you been trying to help resolve some of the ways your clients see their relationship as unfair, and what difference has this made?

- Are there any fairness issues that you have not yet addressed with your client(s) but see as beneficial for future therapeutic work? What has prevented you from addressing these issues so far?

Recognizing Ruptures of Trust

As we have discussed in previous chapters, trust is a fundamental ingredient for family relationships to function and to flourish. One of the responsibilities of the contextual supervisor is to recognize ruptures of trust that the supervisee's clients may be experiencing, as well as potential trust issues clients could experience in the future if change does not occur. The contextual supervisor understands that, regardless of the supervisee's theoretical orientation, it will be difficult to make substantial, sustainable changes within relationships if implications of trustworthiness are not addressed as they relate to clients' problems. Addressing trust can be especially relevant and important when working with couples since it represents a foundational element of creating and sustaining relationships (e.g. Gangamma, Bartle-Haring, & Glebova, 2012). To process implications of trust on therapy processes with a supervisee, consider these questions:

- Can you think of any trust issues that may be currently impairing your clients from having healthy and satisfying relationships?
- What violations of trust have your clients experienced in their family relationships, and in what ways have you been trying to attend to them?
- In what ways, have you noticed your clients behaving toward those who have violated their trust? Have your clients taken any productive steps to begin repairing trust in this relationship?

Exploring Loyalties and Loyalty Conflicts

Family loyalty is a complex concept that underscores many conflicts, and learning how to ask questions about it can be perplexing even to the most seasoned clinicians. For instance, it can be difficult to understand how adult children can continue to feel loyalty to their mother and father even after they have experienced a great deal of emotional pain in these relationships. Using a contextual therapy framework also encourages therapists and supervisors to unify and create greater loyalty and commitment within family relationships in the context of promoting individual health and well-being.

Like Doherty (1995), we believe that therapists have a moral obligation to challenge clients to be committed to their family members and, in turn, hold clients accountable for acting upon those commitments. Of course, these commitments need to be balanced with the importance of respectful, non-toxic interactions. This delicate skill can be developed through seeking contextual-focused supervision, where supervisees can process how to (1) encourage actions that show commitment and (2) honor clients' individual, unique expressions of commitments and responsibilities. As with other systemic models, contextual therapy recognizes that there is a "pull for togetherness" in relationships and a desire to be loyal to a person's family. At times, this means that loyalty to one's family supersedes individual preferences, and it can be tough to decipher how and when to show loyalty. Thus, supervisors should remain mindful of how the supervisees are supporting clients in balancing loyalty to the family and also individual autonomy. In other words, clients can be encouraged to make decisions in relationships freely rather than simply feeling obligated. Healthy expressions of loyalty must also be counterbalanced with healthy and meaningful boundaries.

A contextual supervisor, likewise, has a moral obligation to challenge therapists to find ways to improve the loyalties and commitments that regulate their clients' relationships. In particular, the contextual supervisor should pay close attention to the intersections between loyalties in vertical family relationships (parent and child, grandparent and grandchild) and horizontal family relationships (couples and siblings), as well as how these loyalties impact the family as a whole. Some sample questions to consider asking the supervisee about loyalty include:

- How would you describe the loyalty that this particular client has to their family members? How do people within this family show their commitment to one another?

- What potential loyalty conflicts do you notice in this couple (or family)? How could you address those conflicts to honor all the relationships important to them?

- Have any members of this family experienced any recent violations of loyalty that may be hindering their ability to function and be satisfied in this relationship?

Detecting Entitlement

A contextual supervisor also looks for ways in which entitlement to receive demonstrations of love, care, and trustworthiness acts as a powerful force within relationships and contributes to the constant state of motion of giving and taking within families. Like an ever-changing, exhilarating, and exhausting puzzle, there is a constant rebalancing and restructuring of the expectations that family members have of one another. Entitlement often seems especially prominent in parent-child and couple relationships.

As a reminder, it is up to the individual, couple, or family (not the therapist) to determine what is fair, equal, balanced, and just in their relationships, and supervisors support their supervisees in remaining grounded in this perspective. The supervisor helps to (1) focus the supervisee on the expectations and entitlements that individual clients may have in their relationships and (2) assists the supervisee in recognizing how clients act both constructively and destructively based on these entitlements. Entitlements do not occur in individual vacuums; rather, they are affected by past experiences in relationships and spill over into current expectations, as well. Certainly, a contextual supervisor should raise concerns if any abuse or infidelity may be involved, but clients should be given a level of autonomy to determine what feels balanced in their relationships in the absence of grave harm. A starting place for entitlement-based questions can be found here:

- What do you believe your clients feel entitled to receive in their relationships? Where do you believe that your clients learned what they should expect from their relationships? What experiences in their family or in other previous relationships might have had an impact on these expectations?

- In your client's relationships, are there any that seem balanced and fair (or were fair and balanced in the past)? What is different about these relationships, as opposed to the relationships that seem unbalanced?

- What difference would it make for this couple if they each felt that the contributions of their partner were fair or more equal? What sorts of common expectations do the partners have of each other? In what ways have you been working to balance the expectations that these partners have in their relationship?

Acknowledging Contributions

At times, clinicians can overlook some of the ways their clients may actually be trying to make a positive contribution in their relationships. These represent valuable opportunities that, if missed, can erode the therapeutic relationship and continue contributing to an overall negative narrative in the clients' relationships. Helping supervisees to recognize ways in which family members are contributing (and have contributed) to the overall health of their relationships is valuable to process during supervision consultations. Sometimes the contributions of certain family members may be very small or seem insignificant, but from the contextual tradition of thinking, they should still be acknowledged. Intentions matter.

Clients may get overwhelmed by painful memories and hyper-focus on how family members have failed to show love, care, and loyalty. These negative expectations then cloud their ability to notice attempts to repair injustices or other trustworthy things this person does. This represents another area in which the skill of multidirected partiality is useful. The supervisor encourages the supervisee both to empathize with the person who is hurting and hesitant to trust and also to recognize the contributions of others. The following questions can be used to help supervisees think about how to acknowledge the efforts and contributions of their clients and family members:

- In what ways have you noticed each family member contributing to the overall success of their relationships (even if the contributions may seem insignificant or have gone unrecognized by others)?

- Which family members do you particularly empathize with? What is it about their contributions to their relationships that you personally value? With whom is it hardest to empathize, while acknowledging their efforts? How do you think this has impacted the therapy process so far? How can you broaden your perspective and acknowledge the efforts of other individuals in these relationships?

- Is there a particular perspective inside or outside of the therapy room that deserves more credit and acknowledgment that you have not previously addressed?

Promoting Accountability to Others

One of the very best ways to promote change in family relationships is by promoting accountability in family relationships. In other words, as therapists hold each family member accountable for their actions, the whole family benefits. Similarly, contextual supervisors remain aware of the accountability they have toward their supervisee and the clients. The supervisor gently holds the supervisee accountable for having the courage to empathetically confront clients when needed and help propel them toward change. Sude and Gambrel (2017) also called for trainers and supervisors to model responsible uses of power for their trainees so they can use power that is validating and challenging, but not oppressive, in their work relationships with colleagues and clinical relationships with patients and families.

When feelings of unfairness dominate, families commonly devolve into pointing the finger of blame at others. In reality, however, there are almost always ways that each individual can improve in their role as a mother or father, husband or wife, brother or sister, daughter or son. Although holding clients accountable may feel uncomfortable, supervisors can assist struggling supervisees to have courage when asking difficult questions about how their clients can improve their accountability to one another and imagine creating relationships that are more solid in trustworthiness, loyalty, and justice. Some questions about accountability for supervisees include:

- In what ways, do you believe this family has room to grow, develop, and change? If this family made these changes, what do you think some positive outcomes might be? How does this connect to current goals the family is working on?

- Do any of the individuals within this family seem resistant to or hesitant about making changes discussed in therapy? What do you believe is preventing this person from moving toward change? How do you see this influencing the rest of the family?

- In what ways, have you held each member of this family accountable for their own behavior in their relationships? What seems to be helping? What hasn't helped so far? Who do you think you still need to challenge, and how will you go about holding this individual accountable?

A Springboard for Self-of-the-Therapist Work

Compared to some of the other approaches to family therapy supervision, transgenerational supervision frameworks tend to focus more on helping therapists and therapists-in-training identify pertinent self-of-the-therapist issues. What is included in the concept of self-of-the-therapist issues? Timm and Blow (1999) described self-of-the-therapist work as "the willingness of a therapist or supervisor to participate in a process that requires introspective work on issues in his or her own life that have an impact on the process of therapy in positive and negative ways" (p. 333).

Addressing personal issues that impact how we as clinicians provide therapy (or other health services, for that matter) is essential to the process of clinical growth that distinguishes mediocre therapists from those who excel. Timm and Blow (1999) also called attention to the need for balancing self-of-the-therapist work to include reflection upon how family of origin experiences and historical life events both restrain clinical growth and serve as beneficial resources for work as a clinician. The answer to "How does your personal life impact your ability to do therapy?" is not simple or one-sided.

Like many of the other transgenerational approaches to supervision, such as Bowenian supervision, contextual supervision tends to emphasize helping supervisees make sense of how their own family of origin experiences influence their therapeutic style of working with couples and families (Brooks & Roberto-Forman, 2014). Contextual supervisors help therapists engage in a change process of self-delineation (Boszormenyi-Nagy & Krasner, 1986). Self-delineation includes the ability to understand oneself, self-validate, and separate oneself from others while maintaining meaningful connection (Ducommun-Nagy, 2002). This is essential for developing personal authority and agency in making choices and being willing to be held accountable for them (Brooks & Roberto-Forman, 2014). This type of maturity is necessary for interacting with clients of various ages, genders, and educational backgrounds, and it is also beneficial for maturity in interactions with one's family.

Family of origin experiences can be classified into four relational categories in transgenerational supervision: transgenerational interaction patterns, transgenerationally transmitted cultural beliefs and values, current interactional patterns, and current perceptions and beliefs. The role of the contextual supervisor in this work is to challenge and support supervisees in making sense of these aspects of family life and how they affect their abilities to practice therapy and engage in the process of supervision. According to Brooks and Roberto-Forman (2014):

> Unresolved conflicts create and perpetuate tension, alliances, and coalitions, as well as block give-and-take; create destructive entitlement, triangles, and other side effects in relationships; and therefore become significant supervisory foci. Supervisors help supervisees anticipate how

unresolved [family of origin] issues create potential challenges for maintaining therapeutic differentiation, such as experiencing blind spots, stuckness, or reactivity. (p. 188)

What we have experienced within our families of origin, coupled with experiences in our current relationships, inevitably influences our personal values. The meanings we attribute to our own experiences help form our own beliefs about what fairness, justice, love, trust, and loyalty look like in healthy and unhealthy relationships. Although we must maintain a conscious, critical awareness of our own beliefs and how they influence our therapeutic work, it is impossible to be truly objective and unbiased when working with couples and families. We believe this to be even truer in models such as contextual therapy that are ridden with value-laden constructs such as fairness and justice.

As therapists, we strive to give our clients the freedom to define what is fair, what is loyalty in action, and what actions build up trust. We deeply respect their autonomy and their right to define their own values. However, our humanity predisposes us to (sometimes consciously and sometimes unconsciously) decide whether our clients' perspectives fit with our own or not. The questions we ask, our nonverbal expressions, the goals we write in treatment plans—all are influenced by our own beliefs and values and how we apply those to our interactions with clients. Thus, supervision—whether entered into with a more experienced mentor or peers of a similar clinical level—is essential for therapists in minimizing blind spots and reactivity and maximizing open-mindedness and empathy for all.

However, supervision is not just essential in helping encourage reflection upon family of origin experiences that influence beliefs about fairness and trustworthiness. When was the last time you thought about what you expect to give to your clients or patients and what you expect to receive in return? Fairness expectations guide interactions in personal relationships, as well as in professional relationships. Just as a contextual approach acknowledges an individual's developmental age and circumstances, we also acknowledge the nature of the professional relationship as essential in determining what is fair in terms of creating an equitable system of giving and taking.

For example, it is inappropriate to expect a 5-year-old child to hold primary responsibility in caring for his parent. Similarly, we draw upon the collective wisdom of the psychotherapy field to state that it would likely be inappropriate to expect clients to hold primary responsibility for caring for their therapists' feelings above their own need for personal growth and expression. That type of pattern presents a role reversal since the therapeutic relationship is set up so that the therapist is offering a unique skillset to the client, not the other way around. How much emotional give-and-take you expect from your clients is likely linked to how much you as a therapist disclose about your personal reactions and experiences, and that is certainly linked to an individual therapists' style.

Expectations for balanced giving and taking extend beyond emotional balance in the therapeutic relationship. Another example includes expectations about fair compensation for services offered. Imagine that you are a therapist who sees clients on a sliding-scale-fee basis. If you have the distinct sense that your client is not being honest with you about their family's income and is paying a significantly lower fee than you would deem fair for family therapy, would it not seem plausible that this could breed resentment or frustration? This frustration would likely impact your ability to connect with these clients as they work on therapeutic goals. This leads to an additional benefit of supervision: support in processing perceived injustices that occur within the context of providing therapy and learning to set boundaries that preserve and protect your desired balance of giving and taking with your clients.

PART II: EXPANDED CONTEXTS FOR CONTEXTUAL SUPERVISION

The first section of this chapter emphasized contextual processes relevant to the training and development of couple and family therapists. We believe that the value of contextual supervision extends beyond training for therapists to other types of professionals who work closely with families. One setting which includes a significant number of professionals who work with families can be found in the healthcare system. Healthcare professionals across a wide range of settings are likely to interact with patients' family members, which may spark a desire for additional skills in addressing family dynamics and processing personal reactions brought about by clinical work.

Healthcare presents a natural setting in which basic family therapy skills can contribute to the prevention of, adjustment to, and management of disease within individual and familial contexts. Although this fits most squarely within family therapists' scope of practice to provide ongoing therapeutic support of patients and their families, true family-centered care requires support from a wide range of team members with valuable knowledge to share. Thus, we argue that it is essential for all those team members to be knowledgeable about family dynamics and understand how issues like fairness, loyalty, and accountability play a role in conversations about treatment options, caregiving needs, prognosis, and adjustment to diagnoses.

A contextual supervisor who wishes to offer supervision and consultation for healthcare professionals needs a solid understanding of family therapy skills, as well as (1) practical knowledge about clinical conditions (e.g. diseases, etiologies, treatments) treated within that specific healthcare context and (2) an understanding of operational expectations that affect how care is provided within that specific healthcare setting (e.g. documentation, coordinating care with other providers, job descriptions, scope of practice, etc.). Next, we will briefly describe some ways in which contextual family therapy could be used to facilitate growth in clinical skills in healthcare.

Interprofessional Education

Today's complex healthcare system requires providers and staff to collaborate across multiple disciplines to deliver effective, high-quality patient care. Because communication barriers and differences in philosophical perspectives frequently prevent effective collaboration across professional disciplines, interprofessional education has been suggested as a strategy to improve collaboration and patient care in professional healthcare settings (Reeves, Perrier, Goldman, Freeth, & Zwarenstein, 2013). Reeves and colleagues wrote, "Interprofessional education is defined as an intervention where the members of more than one health or social care profession, or both, learn interactively together, for the explicit purpose of improving interprofessional collaboration or the health/well-being of patients/clients, or both" (p. 2). Interprofessional education could be conducted (1) during formal training prior to

post-graduation employment or (2) during formal and informal training for continuing education throughout a professional career in
healthcare.

For the purpose of improving collaborative communication between
family therapists and medical providers and staff, we propose that semi-
nars or trainings that use the lens of contextual therapy for a medical and
psychosocial audience could be useful in two ways. These trainings have
the potential to increase family therapists' knowledge of medical concepts
and lenses of thinking to plan assessment, treatment, and follow-up.
Additionally, these trainings help improve medical providers' and staff
members' confidence and competence in recognizing and addressing the influence of family dynamics on individual patient outcomes and
care plans.

These interprofessional education sessions could be delivered in a
variety of formats, including half-day workshops, lunch-hour trainings
for staff during a routine clinic meeting, or a single session at a collaborative learning session for continuing education credit. Depending
upon the setting, audience, and time allotment, this type of teaching
could offer some limited opportunities for focused self-reflection (e.g.
family of origin themes and experiences that have influenced one's own
definition of balanced giving and taking and how that impacts beliefs
about patients' caregiving needs) and case consultation for specific
cases (e.g. discussing a current clinical case that highlights a theme
presented during the training).

Orienting and Training Staff to a Family-Centered Model of Care

During their training programs, some medical providers and staff may
have been exposed to practical tips for recognizing, explaining, and
addressing family dynamics that positively and negatively impact patient
care and health outcomes. However, some may lack confidence in
defining their role in addressing problematic family dynamics and may
feel uncertain about how to appropriately refer patients and families to
a family therapist to address underlying dynamics that impede health
and well-being. Thus, orientation for new employees could include
a component of family-centered healthcare that briefly accounts for
a contextual perspective with relevant descriptions for providers and
staff across various levels (e.g. the role of a medical provider vs. a nurse

vs. a care manager). We would recommend this training focus on key behavioral indicators of family-related distress, brief interventions that could be delivered by a variety of staff members, and pragmatic referral partners for patients with more extensive needs. During this type of orientation training, it is likely there would be less emphasis on personal reflection of one's own family of origin issues and more of an emphasis on key skills for recognizing and intervening with problematic family dynamics. However, a training incorporating self-reflection of personal beliefs about fairness, trust, and loyalty could also be beneficial in clarifying values that impact work with patients and families.

Case Consultation

In the healthcare setting, case consultation would likely be the most similar to traditional clinical supervision for therapists. In this type of encounter, a provider (either medical or behavioral health) could request a consultation with a family therapist who has knowledge of contextual therapy. The focus of the consultation would be to discuss points of "stuckness" or confusion with a specific patient or family that are impeding the delivery of quality care. This would most likely include face-to-face or phone discussions about a particular patient, although there could be the opportunity for a joint medical appointment where the therapist could join the medical provider in speaking with the patient and creating a plan of action. This is most likely to occur in an integrated healthcare setting where behavioral healthcare is embedded within the medical clinic. These consultations would likely focus on issues and problems pertaining to that specific case, with some general education about family processes and their relationship to health. Self-reflection work would be anticipated as minimal, depending upon the desire, comfort level, and time allotment of the professional seeking consultation.

Peer Supervision

For healthcare providers who wish to maintain a network of like-minded professionals devoted to family-centered care, peer supervision can be an informal approach to ongoing growth and guidance. Peer supervision can take a variety of formats and could be called by many names, but the general idea is that it provides a structure for clinicians to process the ways in which their cases intersect with their personal beliefs and experiences and offer support to one another as they work with complex patients with challenging circumstances. In the psychotherapy field, this group usually consists of therapists, but the healthcare setting could benefit from routine multidisciplinary meetings with a distinct family-centered care focus. Such meetings could be held as part of or separately from care management meetings that are already included in a clinic's weekly or monthly routine.

Applied within a team-based healthcare setting, these types of group case discussions and ongoing peer supervision could be useful to dive deeper into contextual ideas about fairness, trust, and loyalty and how they apply to patients' health and well-being. Together, the group could develop practical strategies for addressing issues like fairness during limited-time medical appointments. Likewise, the group could discuss specific cases that are treated by multiple providers and staff to strategize how to coordinate care while attending to contextual issues. Although we recognize that contextual issues may not always seem at the forefront of ongoing medical care, we propose that family-centered care would be enhanced by staff receiving training and support from colleagues in addressing how fairness and other concepts drawn from contextual therapy influence patients' experiences within the healthcare system. A team-based approach would provide additional opportunities to activate the resources found in relational ethics in families as they navigate complex health decisions.

REFERENCES

Boszormenyi-Nagy, I. & Krasner, B. R. (1986). *Between give and take: A clinical guide to contextual therapy.* New York, NY: Brunner/Mazel.

Brooks, S. & Roberto-Forman, L. (2014). The transgenerational supervision models. In T. C. Todd & C. L. Storm (Eds.), *The complete systemic supervisor: Context, philosophy and pragmatics.* (2nd ed., pp. 187–207). West Sussex, UK: Wiley.

Doherty, W. J. (1995). *Soul searching: Why psychotherapy must promote moral responsibility.* New York, NY: Basic Books.

Ducommun-Nagy, C. (2002). Contextual therapy. In R. F. Massey & S. D. Massey (Eds.), *Comprehensive handbook of psychotherapy* (Vol. 3, pp. 463–488). New York, NY: John Wiley & Sons.

Gangamma, R., Bartle-Haring, S., & Glebova, T. (2012). A study of contextual therapy theory's relational ethics in couples in therapy. *Family Relations, 61*(5), 825–835.

Reeves, S., Perrier, L., Goldman, J., Freeth, D., & Zwarenstein, M. (2013). Interprofessional education: Effects on professional practice and healthcare outcomes (update). *Cochrane Database of Systemic Reviews, Issue 3*. Art. No. CD002213.

Roberto, L. (2002). The transgenerational supervision models. In T. C. Todd & C. L. Storm (Eds.), *The complete systemic supervisor: Context, philosophy and pragmatics.* (1st ed., pp. 156–172). Lincoln, NE: Authors Choice.

Sude, M. E. & Gambrel, L. E. (2017). A contextual therapy framework for MFT educators: Facilitating trustworthy asymmetrical training relationships. *Journal of Marital and Family Therapy, 43*(4), 617–630.

Timm, T. M. & Blow, A. J. (1999). Self-of-the-therapist work: A balance between removing restraints and identifying resources. *Contemporary Family Therapy, 21*(3), 331–351.

Todd, T. C. & Storm, C. L. (Eds.) (2014). *The complete systemic supervisor: Context, philosophy and pragmatics.* (2nd ed., pp. 187–207). West Sussex, UK: Wiley.

HEALTH-RELATED APPLICATIONS OF CONTEXTUAL THERAPY

Chapter 5

Tailoring the Contextual Framework for Healthcare

This chapter represents a turning point in this book. Thus far, we have spent some time describing the basic underpinnings of contextual therapy as a refresher for therapists who have already learned about it and as a brief guide for those unfamiliar with this model of therapy. Contextual therapy can be practiced in a wide variety of settings and with a broad array of problems; the rest of this book will focus on specific applications within healthcare to help families prevent and manage the many individual and relational demands of illness.

In many ways, this represents uncharted territory. We know of no other authors who have provided an in-depth examination of how to incorporate key principles and concepts from contextual therapy in helping families navigate the healthcare system and adjust to difficulties presented by illness. It is our hope that medical family therapy (MedFT) practitioners and their colleagues will expand their awareness of MedFT-appropriate models to include concepts from a contextual therapy framework. This chapter will (1) build a case for the associations between contextual constructs like relational ethics and health outcomes and experiences in the healthcare system and (2) describe some key recommendations for incorporating a contextual framework in various types of medical settings. The next few chapters will focus on how to apply those associations in working with families with specific types of health problems and provide some illustrative case examples with sample contextual interventions.

WHAT'S RELATIONAL ETHICS GOT TO DO WITH IT? A CONTEXTUAL VIEW ON HEALTH

Boszormenyi-Nagy (1987) recognized that the ideas comprised in contextual therapy can be applied to health and believed strongly that, "Each family member's individual health aspirations become components of the therapeutic contract" (p. 136). Contextual therapists commit themselves to promoting the quality of each one of their clients' lives, not just selecting one individual in the family to support in becoming healthier. This remains a consistent goal, regardless of malfunctions spread across the system or individual complaints (Boszormenyi-Nagy & Krasner, 1986). In short, the contextual therapist is interested in the *complete context* of what everyone in the family system may be experiencing (biologically, psychologically, socially, and spiritually) and how to help each person achieve the best quality of life possible while operating within a contextual framework.

It is impossible to create clear causal distinctions or linear time processes due to the complex interplay of people's life contexts and health experiences. However, for the sake of organization in this next section, we will focus specifically on answering two questions using a contextual lens:

- How do couple and family dynamics impact the presence and process of health problems?
- How do the presence and process of health problems impact the experiences of couples and families?

There is great value in recognizing both perspectives: how contextual constructs impact health and how health impacts contextual experiences. In providing patient care, clinicians must be able to identify times when a health crisis precipitates struggles within the family, but it is also important to recognize deeper roots of problematic behaviors and beliefs that perpetuate poor adjustment to medical diagnosis or interfere with proper disease management. By presenting two sides of this same coin, we hope readers will be able to untangle these threads in their own minds and apply these ideas in clinical cases of their own.

How Contextual Constructs Influence Health

Although the answers to the above two questions are closely intertwined, this first section will describe how a contextual framework can be used to understand how concepts such as trust, loyalty, and fairness influence patients' individual health outcomes. In addition, we will cover how relational dynamics (viewed through the lens of contextual therapy) affect families' adjustment to and coping with various forms of illness. We will describe some general theoretical and research-based ideas in this section, and the following chapters will provide a deeper look at specific illness types using clinical case studies.

What does research show us about the effects of relational ethics on individual health and well-being? Although other researchers have studied the relationships between relational ethics and couples' marital satisfaction, (e.g. Gangamma, Bartle-Haring, & Glebova, 2012), only one published study framed by the lens of contextual therapy has examined the association between relational ethics and physical and mental health symptoms. With a national sample of 632 mid-life, married individuals, Grames, Miller, Robinson, Higgins, and Hinton (2008) demonstrated that participants who reported lower levels of vertical relational ethics in family of origin relationships tended to report higher levels of depression and an increased number of physical health problems. The same association was also found between lower levels of horizontal relational ethics and higher levels of depression and an increased number of physical health problems. This supports ample amounts of research demonstrating a link between poorly managed stress and compromised immune systems (e.g. Reed & Raison, 2016) and stress and detrimental health behaviors such as poor diet and exercise (e.g. Krueger & Chang, 2008). Marital satisfaction mediated the relationships between vertical and horizontal relational ethics and depression and physical health problems. The authors concluded that couples who maintain responsibility for their own actions and offer due consideration to each other are more likely to be satisfied in their marital relationships, which positively affects emotional and physical well-being.

The findings of this study served as a springboard for the first author's (ASH) dissertation, which used contextual therapy to study outcomes related to a specific disease: type 1 diabetes in a sample of young adults. This study, not yet published, examined associations between relational ethics; patient activation of knowledge, skills, and confidence to engage in health management; diabetes self-management behaviors; and health outcomes including HbA1c level, diabetes-related complications, and diabetes-related hospitalizations. Results showed a strong relationship between patient activation and engagement in diabetes self-management behaviors, as well as an indirect relationship between vertical relational ethics, patient activation, diabetes self-management, and number of health problems associated with diabetes. More specifically, participants who reported higher levels of trust and justice, loyalty, and entitlement in their families of origin were more likely to report higher levels of confidence in managing their diabetes, which was associated with better health outcomes.

Together, these two studies suggest that ruptures in relational ethics can potentially lead to an increased risk of poorer mental health and physical health, both in general and with regard to some specific disease outcomes. However, additional research is needed to more clearly define the mechanisms by which this occurs. For example, one question concerns whether the association between relational ethics and health outcomes is mediated by engagement in beneficial or detrimental health behaviors.

Furthermore, the results of AH's dissertation suggest that it may be most important for therapists to guide clients toward questions about how trustworthiness, justice, and loyalty within the family specifically relate to diabetes care (or whatever disease may be most relevant to that particular patient). The general sense of confidence that individuals have in their families' abilities to be reliable and meet their needs may be less important than their confidence in family members to be trustworthy and reliable in helping to manage the practical and socio-emotional demands of a specific illness. Thus, contextual intervention efforts should be tailored to understand relational ethics within the context of the specific illness, as opposed to general well-being for the most improvement in health outcome.

As the driving force behind trust and perceptions of fairness within families, relational ethics is defined by the balance of giving and receiving within family relationships. Thus, relational ethics provides us with one lens through which we can understand how families balance physical and emotional caregiving during times of illness. In cases where the balance of giving and receiving already feels tilted, a health crisis can fuel greater distress and facilitate poorer adjustment to the tasks of disease management and caregiving and support from family members. When trust and loyalty are strained, it can be very difficult to be a patient reliant upon support from others and have faith that one's needs will be met by others. Similarly, it can be difficult for caregivers to make the necessary sacrifices with genuine generosity, as opposed to operating primarily out of a sense of rigid duty.

Relational ethics in the context of health management and caregiving also includes questions about who is responsible for doing the work of caregiving. Difficult as they may be, discussions about caregiving roles often silently include expectations about how caregiving fits into (1) the pre-existing relationship between each potential caregiver and the person needing the caregiving or support and (2) the general life circumstances that affect the time, financial, and energy resources of the potential caregivers. Tensions often arise when caregiving tasks are unfairly placed on the plate of one person or a small group of people when a more just model might include spreading tasks across a pool of people. However, it is also important to keep in mind that the depth and style of caregiving needs fluctuate over time, and the influence of relationships on health is bidirectional, not unidirectional.

How Health Influences Contextual Concepts

From a contextual perspective, the physical health of family members can impact both relational dynamics within the family and the individual's well-being. The demands of physical illness can especially highlight the continual process of give-and-take, which is central to contextual theory. Caregiving for an ill or injured loved one also has a significant impact on the physical, emotional, spiritual, and social well-being of family members (Roth, Fredman, & Haley, 2015). When illness appears, there are often untold expectations regarding how each individual and the family system should respond. These dynamics are intertwined with people's actual experience of a disease or injury and cannot be separated from the actual experience of the illness itself.

Imagine that you became gravely ill from a chronic disease. Who could you count on to take care of you? Who would respond to your suffering? Who would help you with physical tasks if needed? Being able to trust our family members and others whom we are close to in times of trial and hardship is both relationally ethical and a realistic expectation that helps to fulfill our human longing for connection. We want to know that others "have our back" when times get tough and that we will be supported, both physically and emotionally. To manage the effects of inevitable illness, families must be able to trust each other so that they can do the emotionally taxing work of caregiving and decision-making. Our clinical experience has shown us that families who have a genuine interest and concern for each other's health provide significant physical and relational resources during times of health crises.

Just as challenging experiences of illness test the trust we have in others to show us care in the way we need, illness also tests our views of loyalty. Throughout the lifespan, there are periods of relative wellness and periods of illness. It is easier for many families to demonstrate healthy relational behaviors during fair winds and calm seas (times of relative health). However, the unexcepted onslaught of squalls that brings storms (times of illness or injury) are navigated differently by each individual, couple, and family (Schmidt, Sibley, & Dorman, 2016). Without the strong anchor of loving and empathetic family members and friends, health issues can feel isolating, lonely, and insurmountable. A patient whose family struggles to provide empathetic caring can feel threatened by the sense of loss and question their loyalty to him, especially during this time of need. Likewise, family caregivers are called upon to balance loyalty to the sick person and opportunities to care for themselves and attend to other obligations on a daily basis.

In our own clinical work, we have found that our patients often view health-related issues through a lens of fairness. For example, a daughter may say, "It is not fair that my dad was diagnosed with cancer. I do not feel like I can live without him." For families, this perspective of fairness can be understood both in an existential sense and a relational sense. Existential fairness leads us to question the purpose of such suffering, and relational fairness introduces additional questions about what it means for our relationship with the sick person and others in the family.

Much has been written in recent years regarding the importance of meaning-making for highly stressful experiences such as illness, bereavement, and trauma (e.g. Park & George, 2013). As explained by Rutter (1985), "A person's response to any stressor will be influenced by his appraisal of the situation and by his capacity to process the experience, attach meaning to it, and incorporate it into his belief system" (p. 608). We believe that contextual therapy can provide families with the ability to process very difficult situations and to make meaning from situations that may feel existentially unfair but don't have to become additional burdens infused with relational unfairness, as well.

A contextual framework can help guide families through processing both existential and relational fairness considerations. A father could be angry, frustrated, and devastated that his young child has been diagnosed with cancer; he cannot understand why a young, innocent child would suffer such a terrible disease. A wife may question how their family is possibly going to be able to make ends meet now that her husband has been diagnosed with a form of muscular dystrophy and is no longer able to work; she wonders why this sickness has entered their lives at this stage of life where she expected there to be stability. These questions are not easily answered. We believe it is healthy for families to ask questions like "Why?" during the initial adjustment period when a new diagnosis has been delivered and during key transitional or stress points throughout a long-term illness and recovery. However, we also believe it is more beneficial to spend time focusing on the question "How do we move through this?" than seeking a complete, certain answer to the existential question of "Why?" A family's work to move through the difficulties of caregiving, fear, and uncertainty gives meaning to illness and pain, and that narrative becomes richer over time.

A focus on relational ethics helps clinicians and families assess the balance of giving and receiving within the family system. When major health issues arise, a contextual therapist might ask the family, "How will caregiving tasks will be divided up among family members, support staff, and others? How much is the ill person expected to do? How is this decided based upon their physical ability and health status? Does it seem reasonable to all within the family?" When contributions feel imbalanced across the family system, this adds strain to relationships beyond the concerns derived from worries about physical health problems. Illness introduces varying levels of physical and emotional stress, which are amplified within the context of other unhealthy relationship habits and a lack of appreciation for the sacrifices each person makes for the good of the family. On the other hand, families can also be intentional about using the illness to introduce opportunities for gratitude, reflection, and connection.

Our clinical experience has also shown that contributions by the ill person are often overlooked by others (and even ill persons themselves!). One of the most important tasks for contextually minded clinicians is to sincerely acknowledge the contributions of an ill person to the family system, no matter how inconsequential these contributions seem. These contributions could take various obvious and unconventional forms: reducing unnecessary expenses to save money for the family during periods of unemployment, sharing words of wisdom with loved ones, attempting to assist with household tasks as much as he or she is able, and more. This type of acknowledgement serves two purposes. First, it validates and provides credit to the ill person for the effort they are making in their relationships. Second, this helps model for the family an appreciation for all family members' contributions.

One problem that can arise with imbalances in giving and taking concerns how comfortable family members are in sharing their emotions and worries with one another. Patients may withhold sharing their experience with family caregivers out of fear of looking selfish, not being provided with comfort and support, or looking weak. The same can be true for caregivers, who may feel they cannot (or should not) rely on the person who is sick to provide them with support and comfort. Both contribute to imbalances in relationship and may foster resentment and lack of emotional connection. The challenging task for families here is to find ways to seek connection and intimacy during times of illness, as opposed to resorting to distance as a protective mechanism.

As a final point, patients' experiences of family relationships also influence their perception of the medical system. Individuals develop expectations about trustworthiness, loyalty, and fairness within their families. Similar to the influence of family of origin expectations about trustworthiness and fairness on the development of couple relationships, these expectations impact other relationships, such as those between patients and medical providers. Trust and security are essential elements in a treatment relationship for patients with chronic illnesses, and the level of attachment patients feel to providers has been shown to be connected to outcomes such as adherence to medical regimens and patients' perceptions of treatment (Bonds, Camacho, Bell, Duren-Winfield,

Anderson, & Goff, 2004; Brennan, Barnes, Calnan, Corrigan, Dieppe, & Entwistle, 2013; Ciechenowski, Katon, Russo, & Walker, 2001). For example, Bond (2004) found that patients who reported more trust in their medical provider experienced less hassle associated with the demands of illness and higher consistency in completing self-care tasks that helped to maintain their health. Brennan and colleagues (2013) pointed out the importance of trust as a mutual experience for both patients and providers; how much providers trust their patients may influence the types of treatment options they consider and recommend to the patient and the family.

MAKING THE CONTEXTUAL FRAMEWORK USEFUL IN MEDICAL SETTINGS

Ambulatory Care

For those of you who may be unfamiliar with medical settings, ambulatory care is another word that refers to outpatient primary, specialty, or procedural care. The last decade of healthcare reform has placed significant emphasis on improvements in efficiency and comprehensiveness for outpatient, office-based care. Effective preventive care and care management for patients with complex medical and psychosocial needs has become the hallmark of this era's push for meeting the Quadruple Aim of healthcare reform: enhanced patient experience, improved population health, reduced costs, and improved satisfaction for providers and staff (Bodenheimer & Sinsky, 2014).

One component of what has become known as "advanced primary care" is integrating behavioral health services within primary care offices and/or collaborating with mental health providers within the community to coordinate psychosocial care for patients with complex needs (Center for Medicare and Medicaid Services, 2015). These pressures exist within a trend for practices to move away from fee-for-service models that are similar to a hamster running on a wheel without ceasing; in this type of a model, providers are pressured to order more tests, bill more codes, and do more (sometimes unnecessary procedures) to get paid more (Rosenthal, 2017). This system does not account for the complex nuances of individual patients' needs, which is why a proposed solution focuses on helping practices work toward alternative payment models that support a team of multidisciplinary professionals working to support medical providers in providing biopsychosocial care for patients (e.g. Kathol, Butler, McAlpine, & Kane, 2010; Miller, Brown Levey, Payne-Murphy, & Kwan, 2014; Miller, Ross, Davis, Melek, Kathol, & Gordon, 2017).

However, limited time is one of the most common obstacles cited by physicians and staff working to provide patient care in outpatient settings. As McDaniel, Doherty, and Hepworth (2014) stated, "There is a constant drive toward maintaining both efficiency and quality while treating as many patients as possible per day and meeting standards for appropriate documentation" (p. 80). Appointment times are short and based upon the purpose of the appointment. Some clinics even double-book appointment slots as a business practice to improve access to care for patients and generate additional revenue. This means that the challenge of providing psychosocial care and support for patients and families necessitates (1) streamlining clinical processes and selecting which patients can benefit from brief intervention in the outpatient medical setting or should be referred out to longer-term mental health services, (2) learning how to establish rapport quickly and deliver high-impact interventions, and (3) engage in collaborative decision-making and treatment planning with a multidisciplinary team of providers and staff.

As an insight-based model, a contextual framework can be tricky to implement in a time-limited outpatient medical setting. In our experience, the key is to first determine which patients could benefit the most from assessment and intervention with regard to family dynamics and then to creatively weave contextual constructs such as trustworthiness, balanced giving and taking, and perceptions of fairness during inter-actions with these patients. Contextual constructs can be infused into conversations with patients in a variety of ways, including (1) a well-placed question or two during an appointment with a sole medical provider, (2) well-placed questions and a brief follow-up conversation during a joint visit with a medical provider and a behavioral health provider, and (3) more extensive assessment and intervention during scheduled appointments with a behavioral health provider (either embedded in the clinic or within the community).

Oftentimes, keeping it simple is the key. Some examples include:

- A patient with renal failure who is in remission from alcohol addiction experiences significant guilt due to her partner caring for her and meeting most of her financial and physical needs. The therapist helps the patient to create a list (in contextual terms, a ledger) of what she offers to the relationship and what her partner offers to the relationship, and the patient is able to identify meaningful ways she contributes to the relationship as well. Recognition that this list isn't as one-sided as she has perceived alleviates many of her depressive symptoms compounded by guilt.

- A patient who has Parkinson's disease acts as the primary caregiver for his aging mother with early dementia symptoms. He expresses conflicted emotions: primarily frustration with his siblings for not being present to care for their mother and also a need to protect them from the reality of this disease. The therapist helps him reframe the idea of inviting his siblings to be more involved, which opens this patient's mind to considering the idea. She helps him (1) define clearer boundaries for what he wishes to hold himself accountable to do for his mother and how to balance that with caring for his own health, (2) enlist the help of support agencies like home health, and (3) identify how he might like to frame a conversation with his siblings to ask for more assistance.

- During a family care conference for a man in his forties with amyotrophic lateral sclerosis (ALS), tensions arise as two parents discuss whether they should ask their son (a senior in high school) to postpone beginning college in order to remain at home and help care for his dying father. Subsequent discussions with the son reveal mixed feelings: a deep desire to show loyalty to his family by remaining physically close and anger at the injustice of having to put his life on hold for such an unfair disease. The therapist supports the medical provider during joint appointments by ensuring all family members' concerns are heard and all members' attempts to demonstrate love and care are acknowledged as a plan is made for the father's care and family life.

Inpatient Hospitalization

Although some of the same concepts of applying contextual therapy within ambulatory care settings can carry over into inpatient hospitalization, there are also major differences that impact the potential for contextual therapy to be useful in select situations. The amount of time that a patient spends in the hospital varies greatly, from hours in an emergency room to days or even months in a medical, surgical, rehabilitation, or intensive care unit. In general, people who are hospitalized are there because they are acutely sick and their body is in significant distress or they are receiving intensive treatment that cannot be done on an outpatient basis. This means that timing is of the essence when planning how to conduct therapeutic interventions in the hospital. If a heavily sedated patient is on a ventilator in the intensive care unit, that is probably not the best time to begin an in-depth conversation about his or her family's relational ethics and expectations for caregiving after discharge from the hospital. However, family members may signal to the treatment team that they are in distress and struggling to find balance in caregiving roles and self-care, and stabilizing therapeutic interventions may be more helpful for the family than the patient at that point in time.

Since some patients are hospitalized for extended periods of time, this means that there are often additional opportunities for meeting with patients to address problems in family dynamics contributing to patient care or unfulfilled expectations that have led to disappointment and strife. In the hospital, time demands are not dictated so much around appointment slots (as in ambulatory care) but daily schedules of other treating providers and patients' needs for rest and treatment routines. Examples of ways to infuse contextual concepts into conversations with hospitalized patients include:

- A 12-year-old boy with leukemia stays in the hospital for three weeks at a time during his chemotherapy treatments. The therapist meeting with him and his mom helps them process how to balance spending time at the hospital with the son who has cancer while connecting with her other children at home, who have expressed frustration about her absence. They discuss how to involve his other siblings in age-appropriate ways in the patient's care and continue to build opportunities for family connection and fun, even during boring hospital stays.

- A homeless man with a history of heavy alcohol use and limited social support is admitted to the hospital for liver failure. Although

his physicians have encouraged him to consider residential treatment for addiction, he is hesitant to go. The therapist meets with
him to try to understand his hesitation about seeking addiction
treatment and to increase his motivation toward changing his
drinking behaviors. He reports feeling that he spent his life caring
for other people and no one else really wants him to succeed or
is willing to help him out. The therapist helps him create a plan
to forge connections with others in the community who would
support him in seeking treatment and how to set boundaries to
determine when he feels able to show care to others and when he
feels comfortable asking for help from others.

Referrals to Outpatient Psychotherapy

One of the great strengths of contextual therapy is that it can be a
helpful mode of treatment in wide variety of settings. Most traditionally,
it has been implemented as part of traditional outpatient mental health
treatment for individuals, couples, and families. Even in this outpatient
setting, we believe that a healthy collaboration with other professionals
is necessary for effective therapy work with clients when a health problem is a component of individual or relational distress. This could
include diseases that are currently active (e.g. comorbid diabetes and
depression, along with relational tension related to the ways in which
the family rallies around the patient to show support) or those that are
part of the family's history but still have some lingering effects (e.g.
cancer in remission that continues to stress the family's emotional and
cognitive coping skills).

During outpatient therapy without collaboration with medical professionals, the clinician only knows as much about a disease as the
patient is willing to and can directly share. This is also dependent upon
the clinician's ability to intuit the most helpful questions to ask about
symptoms, available treatments, expected course, etc. Asking clients
to sign a release of information to speak with their medical provider
is helpful since it provides the therapist with the most up-to-date information for gaining a better understanding of the intersection between
physical, mental, and social health. It also allows the therapist to share
with the medical providers information about therapy goals, risk and

protective factors that may influence adjustment to the disease, and insight into relevant facts about the patient's life that influence consideration of treatment options. Being located outside the physician's office offers the greatest amount of flexibility in terms of appointment times and scheduling. Even if the therapist is not officially a staff member at a physician's office, this type of collaborative arrangement conveys a sense of whole-person healthcare and stimulates multifaceted questions about biopsychosocial-spiritual components of health.

Patient and Family Support Groups

Contextual therapists are trained to assess and address unique, interacting perspectives and background context of individuals within a family. This core skill makes them uniquely positioned to facilitate patient and family support groups. Support groups are often structured around common issues (e.g. diabetes management, depression, or substance use disorders), and they offer a setting in which patients can feel understood and validated in a way that is not always achieved in individual psychotherapy with a therapist. Support groups come in a wide variety of formats and can be designed for patients and caregivers. Groups offer the chance to connect with others, openly share emotional burdens and concerns, and learn coping skills from others facing a similar disease or constellation of symptoms (Delisle, Gumuchian, Rice, Levis, Kloda, Körner, & Thombs, 2017).

Contextually informed support groups for patients and family members can provide a valuable framework for helping group members make sense of underlying reasons—factual, psychological, interactional, or relationally ethical—for distress in the context of the disease. Contextually informed groups offer opportunities for the facilitating clinician and other group members to validate perspectives shared and offer gentle suggestions and education about additional perspectives or coping behaviors that could lead to empowerment and hope instead of despair and helplessness. Support groups facilitated through a contextual therapy lens can also help participants to recognize how others also may be experiencing fairness issues in their relationships, which can help to normalize even some of the most difficult circumstances that individuals, couples, and families may be facing.

The challenge, for the contextually minded group facilitator, is to reflect what patients say and offer education without using jargon unique to the contextual perspective. For example, it would not be wise to say, "It sounds like your family has a real problem with relational ethics right now" or "Today, we are going to learn how to understand your life according to the four dimensions of contextual therapy." Group members would be likely to look at you with confused, wary stares and move on to the next topic. Instead, think of ways to tie in the underlying constructs of contextual therapy based on common experiences that are shared in the group. Some examples include:

- Describing that healthy families find a way to balance how they show *and* receive care and support over time and asking how others in the group are working to develop that balance in their own families
- Highlighting areas of imbalance as you hear that theme raised and asking questions like, "How does that impact the sense of unity and teamwork you have in your family?" and "What is a small change that might help you feel like your family is working a little better as a team to address this issue?"

Operationally speaking, there are various ways in which contextually informed support groups for patients and families can be designed. For therapists who work within a medical setting, the therapist could recruit patients from a given clinic or hospital setting to join a group that is focused on a particular condition. For therapists who work in a more traditional mental health setting, the therapist could approach a local organization related to the disease (e.g. Alzheimer's Association) or the leadership of a local clinic or hospital system about contracting to begin a group designed to meet the needs of patients and fill a gap that exists. When designing the structure of the group, the facilitator must decide whether the group will be open or closed, time-limited or operating indefinitely; there are merits to each approach. It may also be helpful to consider adding a co-facilitator or regular guest speakers who can share education and answer questions more related to medical concerns, so we recommend considering healthcare professionals such as medical providers, nurses, clinical pharmacists, physical therapists, occupational therapists, and speech language pathologists as partners in the facilitation process to offer a robust array of resources and information.

RATION TO MEET MULTIDIMENSIONAL NEEDS

Perhaps the most significant barrier to using a contextual framework within the healthcare system pertains to the perceived complexity of contextual constructs. Not surprisingly, words like "relational ethics" and "destructive entitlement" have not made their way into the medical vernacular used in diagnosis and note taking. Thus, a major challenge for contextually trained clinicians is to learn how to convey the underlying themes of contextual constructs in a way that their non-therapy-trained colleagues can digest and intervene accordingly.

In general, behavioral health providers who work in medical settings must learn to adopt a shared language with their medical colleagues as they discuss problems and plans for treating patients. Generally, medical professionals report a desire to receive pragmatic communication from therapists regarding assessment, treatment, and specific recommendations for the physician (McDaniel, Doherty, & Hepworth, 2014). Rather than helping to enhance care coordination, therapeutic jargon serves as a barrier to multidisciplinary collaboration between medically trained and therapeutically trained clinicians. Therefore, it is important to have a good sense of how to explain contextual concepts in a coherent, organized way that makes sense to patients, their family members, and their entire treatment team.

It can be difficult to describe key components of contextual therapy in a clear, pragmatic manner, but we have a few recommendations based upon our years of experience creatively implementing contextual therapy in medical settings. Here are a few of our top tips:

- Connecting psychotherapy-related assessment and goals is most helpful to medically oriented colleagues when connected to specific symptoms that can be included in comprehensive treatment. For example, you could say, "This patient feels like things are really unstable in her family right now as she and her siblings try to decide how best to care for their mother. She has reported experiencing significant anxiety and stress about the situation, which makes it hard for her to sleep at night due to racing thoughts and an inability to relax. She also experiences depressive symptoms like feelings of hopelessness and fatigue, but she did not report suicidal thoughts. We are going to work on managing expectations of her siblings and focusing how to make some small steps toward a plan for caring for her mom that feels shared among the siblings. I am also planning to teach her some sleep hygiene techniques to see if that helps reduce some of the stress about sleep." Essentially, a successful therapist communicates with physicians by balancing (1) a description of psychosocial components surrounding a presenting problem and (2) connecting back to relevant symptoms that the treating medical provider would like addressed, as well.

- "Relational ethics" is not a word you are likely to find helpful to use with medical colleagues unless you wish to watch their eyes glaze over. Rather, the underlying concepts can be described if a provider is interested in collaborating with you to understand underlying problems leading to a patient's concerns or symptoms. One phrase that is less jargon-prone and still expresses the idea of relational ethics could include "balance of giving and receiving from relationships." Discussions can also be relatively easily framed in terms of a patient's expectations about whose job it is to give, under what circumstances, and how to earn trust. Give an example of imbalance in the patient's life to help make the concept more tangible.

- Providers from various disciplines, psychotherapeutically oriented and otherwise, can look for ways to ask patients about their expectations for how family members should show them loyalty during a health problem, how to earn and maintain trustworthiness, and how those beliefs play a role in their physical, mental, social, emotional, and spiritual well-being. Although it takes some practice, it is possible to include these questions during brief encounters by listening for opportunities to inquire about family dynamics that present strength and connection, as well as family dynamics that contribute to tension and stress. These questions provide a foundation for team-based discussions about how to help patients manage the influence of family on their health.

Although contextual therapy has much to offer in the specialty mental health field, there are many components of underlying themes and goals from a contextual framework that can be incorporated into other healthcare settings for individuals, couples, and families. Creativity, simple wording, and intentional examples are essential in the process of applying the contextual framework in the medical system with non-therapy colleagues. In the next several chapters, we will cover specific ways in which contextual therapy constructs intersect with various types of illness trajectories, attending to the role of multiple types of health professionals on the team.

REFERENCES

Bodenheimer, T. & Sinsky, C. (2014). From triple to quadruple aim: Care of the patient requires care of the provider. *Annuals of Family Medicine, 12*(6), 573–576.

Bonds, D. E., Camacho, F., Bell, R. A., Duren-Winfield, V. T., Anderson, R. T., & Goff, D. C. (2004). The association of patient trust and self-care among patients with diabetes mellitus. *BMC Family Practice, 5*(26).

Boszormenyi-Nagy, I. (1987). *Foundations of contextual therapy: Collected papers of Ivan Boszormenyi-Nagy, MD.* New York: Brunner/Mazel.

Boszormenyi-Nagy, I. & Krasner, B. R. (1986). Between give and take: A clinical guide to contextual therapy. New York, NY: Brunner/Mazel.

Brennan, N., Barnes, R., Calnan, M., Corrigan, O., Dieppe, P., & Entwistle, V. (2013). Trust in the health-care provider-patient relationship: A systematic mapping of the evidence base. *International Journal for Quality in Health Care, 25*(6), 682–688.

Center for Medicare and Medicaid Services (2015). Advanced primary care initiatives. Retrieved February 9, 2017 from https://innovation.cms.gov/initiatives/Advanced-Primary-Care/

Ciechanowski, P. S., Katon, W. J., Russo, J. E., & Walker, E. A. (2001). The patient-provider relationship: Attachment theory and adherence to treatment in diabetes. *American Journal of Psychiatry, 158,* 29–35.

Delisle, V.C., Gumuchian, S. T., Rice, D. B., Levis, A. W., Kloda, L. A., Körner, A., & Thombs, B. D. (2017). Perceived benefits and factors that influence the ability to establish and maintain patient support groups in rare diseases: A scoping review. *The Patient—Patient-Centered Outcomes Research, 10*(3), 283–293.

Gangamma, R., Bartle-Haring, S., & Glebova, T. (2012). A study of contextual therapy theory's relational ethics in couples in therapy. *Family Relations, 61*(5), 825–835.

Grames, H. A., Miller, R. B., Robinson, W. D., Higgins, D. J., Hinton, W. J. (2008). A test of contextual theory: The relationship between relational ethics, marital satisfaction, health problems, and depression. *Contemporary Family Therapy, 30, 183–198.*

Kathol, R. G., Butler, M., McAlpine, D., & Kane, R. L. (2010). Barriers to physical and mental condition integrated service delivery. *Psychosomatic Medicine, 72,* 511–518.

Krueger, P. M. & Chang, V. W. (2008). Being poor and coping with stress: Health behaviors and the risk of death. *American Public Health, 98*(5), 889–896.

McDaniel, S. H., Doherty, W. J., & Hepworth, J. (2014). *Medical family therapy and integrated care* (2nd ed.). Washington, DC: American Psychological Association.

Miller, B. F., Brown Levey, S. M., Payne-Murphy, J. C., & Kwan, B. M. (2014). Outlining the scope of behavioral health practice in integrated primary care: Dispelling the myth of the one-trick mental health pony. *Families, Systems, and Health, 32*(3), 338–343.

Miller, B. F., Ross, K. M., Davis, M. M., Melek, S. P., Kathol, R., & Gordon, P. (2017). Payment reform in the patient-centered medical home: Enabling and sustaining integrated behavioral health care. *American Psychologist, 72*(1), 55–68.

Park, C. L. & George, L. S. (2013). Assessing meaning and meaning making in the context of stressful life events: Measurement tools and approaches. *Journal of Positive Psychology, 8*, 6, 483–504.

Reed, R. G. & Raison, C. L. (2016). Stress and the immune system. In C. Esser (Ed.), *Environmental influences on the immune system* (pp. 97–126). Vienna: Springer.

Rosenthal, E. (2017). *An American sickness: How healthcare became big business and how you can take it back.* New York, NY: Penguin Press.

Roth, D. L., Fredman, L., & Haley, W. (2015). Informal caregiving and its impact on health: A reappraisal from population-based studies. *The Gerontologist, 55*(2), 309–319.

Rutter, M. (1985). Resilience in the face of adversity: Protective factors and resistance to psychiatric disorder. *British Journal of Psychiatry, 147*, 598–611.

Schmidt, A. E., Sibley, D. S., & Dorman, C. (2016, November 29th). Fair winds and squalls: The health impact of family legacies across the lifespan [Blog post]. Retrieved February 25, 2018 from www.cfha.net/blogpost/753286/263378/ Fair-Winds-and-Squalls-The-Health-Impact-of-Family-Legacies-Across-the-Lifespan

Chapter 6

The Crisis is Real

Demands of Acute Conditions

Part of the mystery surrounding health problems is due to the seemingly endless variety of presentations of symptoms and problems with functioning. Rolland (1994) developed a psychosocial typology of diseases that classifies health problems according to their onset (acute vs. gradual), course (progressive vs. constant vs. relapsing), outcome (nonfatal vs. shortened lifespan or sudden death vs. fatal), and degree of incapacitation (none vs. mild vs. moderate vs. severe). Although there are certainly many ways to categorize the types of health problems that face families across their lifespans, this particular typology shines a light on some of the key areas which we have found families to refer to when grappling with feelings of existential or relational unfairness. In particular, the type of onset of symptoms seems to play a particularly important role in families' abilities to adjust to diseases and organize resources and support.

With chronic diseases, symptoms can have an insidious start that is difficult to identify with a clear beginning, and illness can linger for long, sometimes unknown, periods of time. Other times, these symptoms seem to appear from out of nowhere and can be tied to a particular event such as an accident, injury, or acute medical event. The suddenness of these acute health problems places additional strain on patients and families who face the necessity of making decisions quickly, often having a limited understanding at the time of the underlying factors of the problem or an expected prognosis. In this chapter, we will describe key challenges associated with illnesses that be described as having an acute onset and use a case study to illustrate some ways to conceptualize contextual concepts such as trustworthiness, balanced giving-and-taking, and loyalty as related to this family's adjustment to a series of strokes.

CHALLENGES OF ACUTE ILLNESS

As noted by Rolland (1994), illnesses with an acute onset are not necessarily different biologically from those with a gradual onset. Rather, what sets illnesses with an acute onset apart from others is that symptoms have a sudden presentation and are noticed rapidly, either by the patient or others around them. These problems often require a trip to the emergency department or a stay in the hospital, short or extended in length. Examples of acute health problems include heart attacks, strokes, asthma attacks, meningitis, spinal cord injuries, traumatic brain injuries, and burns. This may sound simple, but there are some complexities to consider. Acute conditions can be of a short duration (like food poisoning) or can have consequences that last for some time (like a stroke, for example). It is also important to consider that some chronic conditions, such as congestive heart failure, include periods of acute exacerbation with increased fatigue and difficulty breathing when lying down.

With such a sudden change in health state, patients and their families are forced to rapidly make emotional and practical changes in a very short, compartmentalized period of time. These are similar to the skills needed during crisis management (Rolland, 1994). The decisions needing to be made can feel overwhelming and debilitating, and some families are too shocked by the sudden crisis to activate the resources they need to cope with this trial. Others, however, thrive in this type of quick-thinking environment and are able to bond together to make difficult decisions in unity and peace. What is the difference?

Contextually speaking, there are many possibilities. One is that a crisis can put previous relational problems into perspective and "shake things up," perhaps into a better balance than they were before. Another possibility is that if a family has been divided before a health crisis, the individual members may feel extra guarded during the crisis and be increasingly attentive to any signs of unfairness or untrustworthiness.

As you can imagine, this is likely to make the situation feel ev
unbearable and stressful.

Contextual Roots of Decision-Making and Caregiving

The decisions needing to be made by the family and the emotional and
practical resources required depend on a variety of factors, such as the
level of impairment, the expected course of the disease, and the age of
onset. These factors play into the type of caregiving the patient will
need, and practical and financial limitations certainly influence whether
the family is able to provide care at home or the patient will need to stay
somewhere like a nursing facility for a period of time. Although sometimes it may be impossible for families to provide care at home, we have
seen several families' struggles within their relationships lead to a closed-
mindedness to the option of in-home caregiving, regardless of any
practical limitations. However, we also have seen other families use an
acute health crisis as an opportunity to demonstrate love and care for an
ill family member and repair old emotional wounds.

Given the circumstances of an acute health crisis, families need to
quickly reorganize themselves to accommodate the needs of the patient.
This can lead to feelings of undue burden on one or several members
if it is perceived that some other people within the family are not
reorganizing their own lives while others are. Left unattended, these
types of perceptions can lead to longer-term feelings of resentment,
hurt, and anger. Talking to a person in this type of situation, you might
hear them say something like, "Why is it that I have to take time off work
to deal with this? My sister seems to continue her life like nothing ever
happened. It is like she thinks her responsibilities are more important
than mine, and she has no idea how much I am sacrificing to be here."
In this type of situation, a contextually minded clinician working with
the family could work to help all family members (1) understand why
certain members are less willing or able to shift their daily routines and
resources to accommodate increased caregiving and (2) negotiate
a mutually satisfying arrangement that honors what each individual
family member is actually able to contribute to the system in crisis.
Remember from our initial chapters on fairness: equal is not the same
as equitable.

Next, a case study will be used to describe the story of one couple who faced a series of acute illness events. We will use this story to illustrate how one healthcare team was able to infuse elements from contextual therapy in the treatment of this patient and his loved ones. We will highlight ways in which a therapist and medical provider collaborated to promote healing in the midst of greater personal suffering and uncertainty.

CASE STUDY 6.1

Craig and Stacy met through some mutual friends and quickly fell in love. They became engaged about a year ago, and this is where their story departs from that of many couples they know. One month after becoming engaged, their wedding planning was put on hold when Craig experienced his first stroke at the age of 49. After spending some time in a rehabilitation unit, Craig still experienced difficulties with balance that required the use of a walker. Although he retained his speech and was not permanently paralyzed, Craig developed mild depression following the stroke. He felt doubtful about the possibility of recovery and embarrassed about his inability to "walk like a normal person." However, he tried to "just be positive" and found that spending time with his adult children and grandchildren lifted his mood. Unfortunately, six months later, he suffered a second stroke.

This second stroke interfered even more with his balance and move-ment, and it also led to significant problems with his short-term memory. His difficulties during daily conversations led to frustration for him and others, and he felt too ashamed to try to start conversations with those outside his closest family members. In turn, Craig's depressive symptoms rocketed into the moderate-severe range, including loss of appetite, strong feelings of hopelessness, and passive suicidal thoughts about wishing he were no longer alive. With intensive home-based physical therapy, Craig regained enough strength and coordination to complete basic tasks such as dressing and bathing himself with some minor accommodations to their home. However, his fear of falling prevented him from feeling motivated to work on household chores and projects.

Since he was unable to drive, he relied on Stacy for getting to appointments and running errands. Despite insurance benefits that would allow for significant in-home assistance, Craig's pride prevented him from accepting help from people he did not trust. In fact, he stated repeatedly that "Stacy is the only one who knows how to take care of me." For several months, Stacy stayed at home with Craig during the day and worked full time at a local grocery store with night shifts.

Stacy shouldered a lot of responsibility within the family as the sole financial provider and primary caregiver for Craig. Because she spent most of her time working, taking Craig to medical appointments, or tending to household tasks, she felt she had zero time to do things she enjoys and could not spend time with other family members or friends who live across town. Overwhelmed and burdened but embarrassed to ask for help, she slowly grew to resent Craig and his poor health for filling her with so much pain and guilt and fear. She was uncertain whether to move forward with wedding plans but also could not imagine life without Craig. She was stuck.

Fifteen years ago, Stacy's father died due to a stroke that was not treated in time, and she always felt guilty that she did not have the chance to care for her aging father and return the love he showed her as a child. She thought of Craig's stroke as "an opportunity to show someone I love how much I'm willing to do for them." However, Stacy struggled to be as kind and emotionally grounded as she wished to be most days, which triggered feelings of guilt and anger at herself. She reported that her brain was "always buzzing" and she had trouble falling asleep, despite being physically exhausted. Eating became one of her few sources of comfort; much to her dismay, she gained 25 pounds in four months.

At a follow-up appointment to address post-stroke recovery, Craig's family physician made a referral for Craig and Stacy to meet with a behavioral health provider (DS). When I met with Craig and Stacy, I learned that prior to Craig's strokes, he was an executive for a nationwide trucking company where he had worked for 35 years. After his second stroke, Craig lost his ability to drive, which eliminated one of his greatest passions in life. He found joy and freedom in driving on open highways, and his sense of adventure inspired him to take any job that required driving across the country. He explained, "I used to manage well over 500 drivers across the country, and now I feel worthless. I have let everyone down. This is not fair! I am only 57 years old, and now I have no way to support my family aside from the little I get from disability. It just isn't enough. I'm a drain on them, just taking up time and money."

When I asked how she feels about what Craig just said, Stacy shrugged. With a quiet sigh and an exasperated tone, she explained that she continually feels anxious about money, Craig's health, and "just about everything else. It's too much." She gave another tired sigh and said she's not sure they'll ever feel caught up. The hopelessness in the air was palpable, and the couple sat in chairs on opposite sides of the room, barely looking at one another.

Conceptualizing the Case

What to do in a situation like this? We will look at this case through the lens of contextual therapy to explore contextual constructs we see at play. First, let us conduct an assessment of what we know so far and organize it according to the four dimensions of a contextual framework.

Factually, Craig and Stacy were engaged to be married and are cohabiting, which intertwined various relational and financial aspects of their lives. Craig suffered several strokes that led to memory and physical movement problems, as well as changes in his general mood. Craig previously worked in a manager-level position but is now unemployed and relies on disability for a small amount of income. Stacy's own health problems included a family history of stroke and personal weight gained as a result of inactivity and emotional overeating.

Psychologically, Craig's sense of inadequacy to contribute financially to his family led to concerns about his own self-worth, and he felt guilt over being a burden to others. With significant medical bills and limited income, money had become the currency in this family to define any positive contribution. Stacy's guilt over not being present at the time of her father's death also weighed her down and certainly impacted her thoughts about the necessity of doing all she could to support Craig in his post-stroke recovery.

Transactionally, Craig and Stacy were more physically interdependent than they had been previously in their relationship since Stacy provided much day-to-day and practical support to Craig. However, this intense caregiving and silently mourning the life they had planned for stood in the way of their emotional closeness. They each felt lonely and isolated in their grief over the loss of the healthy life together they had hoped for.

Concerning *relational ethics*, Craig and Stacy were struggling with both relational and existential fairness. In an existential sense, they were grieving the loss of the married life they had anticipated just a few short months ago, and they had been confronted with their own mortality. Both felt they had been dealt a "short hand" in life, with Craig's physical, mental, and socioemotional capacity limited by strokes and Stacy's time and energy constrained by caregiving duties. Relationally, Stacy struggled to balance two parts of her: one that logically understood Craig's need for additional help and his limited capacity to help around the house, and another part that felt the weight of unfairness that she had to take on so many duties amidst her own stress and grief. She believed that Craig could no longer do any household duties or work and took significant burdens upon herself; however, her resentment poisoned her openness to emotional and physical intimacy with Craig.

What to do with all this information as a contextually minded clinician? A few questions come to mind that may help to shine some light on a deeper context of Craig and Stacy's situation and how to help. Some sample curiosities include:

- Did a sense of unfairness and imbalance in the relationship exist before Craig's health problems, or are these newer feelings that have arisen?

- How do Craig and Stacy's support system impact their coping? Which friends and family members help alleviate some of their burdens and provide practical and emotional support at this time? Which friends or family seem to heighten their anxiety about the unfairness of the situation by making unhelpful comments or introducing unrealistic expectations?

- How did the suddenness of the stroke symptoms, with no time to prepare physically or emotionally, impact their ability to cope? How was this experience similar to or different from health problems they have watched other friends or family members endure?

Planning Interventions

Once you understand more about the context of Craig and Stacy's
suffering, you can make a plan for how to intervene. Craig and Stacy
may have many goals (financial, health-related, etc.) that they hope to
achieve, but it may be helpful to focus initially on how to help this
couple develop their teamwork skills. It is hard to survive a crisis when
you do not have a team mindset, and it is hard to create a good team
without security and trustworthiness, loyalty to a common goal, and a
commitment to fairness. Depending upon the security of the relational
ethics foundation that Craig and Stacy had before the strokes, this
process may require significant effort, especially if their partnership was
strained prior to the health problems.

There are many traps that could derail the work that families need to
do to manage an acute health problem, and as a clinician, awareness of
these traps is essential. For example, if there is a long history of damaged
relational ethics, this family could spiral into chaos, rehashing previous
hurts and breakdowns in trust in a way that keeps them from working
toward healing. Although it is essential to understand the context
of various family members' perspectives and roles, one key job of the
clinician is to help families dealing with an acute health problem
to filter through (1) what is important to address at this moment to
respond to immediate needs and (2) what would be best served to wait
to address at a time where the family is more stable and able to devote
more energy to resolution. Unproductive, extended conversations about
past wrongs committed are unlikely to be satisfying or helpful during
times when fear, uncertainty, and high-stakes decision-making prevail.
Rather, the focus (during a crisis) must be on finding solutions to
problems at hand and trying to draw upon the resources that each
person in the family brings to the table.

Now that we have organized our assessment of what we know so
far, let us consider what we might do with this information in terms of
enacting some interventions with Craig and Stacy. Indeed, questions
that clinicians ask can serve various purposes, ranging from helping the
clinician orient himself to the client's experience to provoking some
sort of reflection and therapeutic change (Tomm, 1998). For a family
like Craig and Stacy's experiencing a health crisis, the general idea is to
help answer the contextually framed questions, "In the context of this

terrible, unpredictable health event, how can you bond together to use this crisis for good? How can you use this time to grow your commitment to one another? How can you honor the resources you both bring to help work toward resolving problems and create a new balance of giving and receiving?"

One excellent starting place could include coordinating with Craig's medical providers to more fully understand his physical limitations at this time and what he could reasonably do around the house. One assumption of contextual therapy is that people function best when they are able to be productive in providing something to others and are acknowledged for their contributions, no matter how small they seem. However, in the context of a life-changing medical event, it's important to work with medical staff to maintain realistic expectations that will not hinder healing and recovery. Although Craig's depression has tried to convince him that he is a worthless drain on his family's finances and energy, a contextually minded clinician could (1) sincerely convey to Craig that, regardless of his health status, he has something to share with his family and his community and (2) help coach Craig into creating a list of concrete ways in which he could put those talents and resources into action.

In this case, Craig decided he would commit to filling out disability paperwork and not leaving that for Stacy to do, cutting coupons from the weekly newspaper to help save money at the grocery store, and folding laundry as it came out of the dryer. He also committed to telling Stacy "thank you" at least once a day to help increase her awareness of his appreciation for her sacrifices, and he set a goal of asking about her day instead of just complaining about his. Finally, he aimed to find a stroke support group to attend so he could "learn what other people have done to adjust and be a good friend to someone who's gone through the same thing." Upon writing a half-page list of things he could do, even with his post-stroke difficulties, Craig seemed surprised. He slowly began to realize that he could do more than he thought, and this seemed to help increase his confidence in himself and his abilities and assuage his guilt over "stressing Stacy out all the time."

Another intervention to help strengthen Craig and Stacy's teamwork skills in dealing with this health crisis focused on helping them reflect upon a previous struggle that they successfully resolved together. A solution-oriented line of questioning with a contextual flair aimed to help Craig and Stacy consider a time in which they faced a significant challenge and were able to work through it together in a way that showed them how to trust one another and put their resources into action. Follow-up questions included: "Craig, what was it that Stacy did to show you that you were both working toward a common goal?" and "Stacy, how did Craig's appreciation of how hard you were working impact your thinking about the future you want to have with him?" Although these may seem like run-of-the-mill therapeutic questions, a contextual framework would encourage the therapist to consider how these responses would influence overall perceptions for Craig and Stacy in terms of fairness in giving-and-taking, trustworthiness, and loyalty to one another and how their changes might impact others in their family and friend systems.

Another contextually framed intervention focused on helping Craig and Stacy to consider tangible, practical ways in which they could demonstrate appreciation for one another's contributions, no matter how small.

In many cases, it is helpful to create a written ledger for each person in order to describe expectations and commitments. A ledger includes both entitlements to receive and obligations to give in a relationship, and what is included varies from relationship to relationship. What could this actually look like in clinical practice? In one column, write what that person expects to receive from his or her partner to help their relationship feel more solid and what he/she will give to the relationship. Although it is impossible to capture all the elements of giving-and-taking in a relationship, this simple exercise has the potential to spark conversation about what is considered fair and just and how this ledger changes with mental, physical, and relational health. Ledgers of giving-and-taking do not remain chiseled in stone; they are fluid, ever-changing agreements that need flexibility to adjust to life's circumstances.

For example, Stacy's ledger in her relationship with Craig might initially have looked like Table 6.1.

Upon reviewing the ledger, the therapist would likely note that the giving and receiving appears to be unbalanced. Hence, the interventions previously mentioned would have served to help balance the ledger and even out the giving and receiving as Craig committed to some practical household tasks that would reduce the burden on Stacy and seek

Table 6.1 *Ledger*

Giving	Receiving
Working full time to provide for the family	Craig occasionally thanks her for her sacrifice to work full time and help care for him
Preparing breakfast and dinner for the family	Craig hugs her often and holds her hand, which gives her a sense of comfort
Driving Craig to doctors' appointments and for needed errands	
Providing a listening ear and encouraging words to Craig during days when he feels depressed or angry	
Doing all laundry for the family, multiple days of the week	
Cleaning the house, grocery shopping, paying bills	

emotional support from additional people. A more balanced ledger provides a foundation for loyalty to one another and trust in a partnership to meet common goals and care for each other's needs.

Key Learning Points

In summary, acute health events are about helping families gain some insight into how past circumstances influence current coping trends, and keep a primary focus on how to maintain teamwork and partnership through a crisis. Regardless of physical ability, all people need to feel recognized for what skills and resources they share with their families and their community. Acute health problems are not an excuse for letting the balance of giving-and-taking become one-sided, but it will likely require some creative thinking about how to redefine contributions. Persons with significant physical or mental impairment may need some coaching to identify other ways in which they can give help and comfort to their family members, and clinicians working with these patients and their families must maintain a profound, sincere belief in the worth and contribution of these patients.

REFERENCES

Rolland, J. S. (1994). *Families, illness, and disability: An integrative treatment model.* New York, NY: Basic Books.

Tomm, K. (1998). Interventive interviewing: Part III. Intending to ask lineal, circular, strategic, or reflexive questions? *Family Process, 27*(1), 1–15.

Chapter 7

It Never Ends

Chronic Disease Challenges

The difficulty of an acute disease stems from its sudden onset forcing quick adjustment, whereas the difficulty of a chronic disease stems from the need for long-term adjustment and a variety of health problems that arise over time. As in the previous chapter pertaining to acute illnesses, we will describe here key challenges associated with chronic diseases. A case study will illustrate some ways to conceptualize contextual concepts such as trustworthiness, balanced giving and receiving, and loyalty as related to a family's adjustment of an adolescent son being diagnosed with type 1 diabetes.

CHALLENGES OF CHRONIC DISEASE

According to the World Health Organization (2017), chronic diseases generally progress slowly and have a long duration. They are typically non-communicable, meaning that they are not passed from person to person. Rather, a variety of genetic and environmental risk factors can lead to the development of symptoms and diagnosis of a chronic disease. Some examples include types 1 and 2 diabetes, asthma, chronic obstructive pulmonary diseases (COPD), and various forms of cancer. With impressive medical advances in the last century, life expectancies are now extended for those who would have almost certainly died earlier. However, this prolonged life is often accompanied by prolonged challenges associated with long-term treatment and medical surveillance (Turner & Kelly, 2000).

The element of time becomes an important concept for the family of a patient with a chronic disease. According to Rolland (1997), "Family members adapt best when they understand the strengths and vulnerabilities connected to past family experiences and legacies they bring to a serious illness and, at the same time, have a useful way to think into the future taking the illness and these prior experiences into account" (p. 141). As with any health problem, it is important to recognize that the diagnosis of a chronic health condition does not exist in isolation from other life cycle and psychosocial context, nor does it only influence the individual carrying the diagnosis.

Ready or not, the diagnosis of a chronic disease forces entrance into a new reality for patients with chronic diseases and their families. Some patients with a new onset or a history of depression, anxiety, or insomnia may find their symptoms heightened during stages of adjustment to a chronic physical disease like diabetes (Chasens & Luyster, 2016; Renn, Feliciano, & Segal, 2011; Smith et al., 2013). There are many hypotheses why, including psychological burden of disease management leading to distress and shared underlying biological and behavioral mechanisms (Holt, Groot, & Golden, 2014). Others may experience a new onset of mental health disorder symptoms as a response to the stress associated with chronic disease care management. The same can be true for caregivers of those with chronic health conditions. Thus, treatment of chronic health conditions should include ongoing inquiry into cognitive, emotional, social, and spiritual coping strategies used by patients and their families and how those coping strategies enhance or detract from their quality of life.

With this new reality comes a mourning of previous health and routines and living with anticipation of loss—loss of control over some bodily functions, loss of former roles, loss of identity as a healthy person, loss of previous routines and life rhythms, and even loss of life in some cases. Families must mourn the loss of the life they had as a family unit before the disease. Many patients experience changes in the role they fill in the family; many patients with whom we have worked over the years have struggled with the idea of no longer being "the strong one" and succumbing to the "patient" role. For these individuals, it can be difficult to accept their dependence upon the care and assistance of others when the illness reaches a stage where that is required. Especially with life-threatening or progressive diseases, families must learn to live with "death over their shoulder" (Rolland, 1994, p. 175), and it takes energy and resourcefulness to balance awareness of the fragility of life with engagement in everyday activities.

Ambivalence about how to cope with symptoms and side effects of treatment and uncertainty about potential outcomes also seem to be par for the course with chronic diseases. Patients and family members can be unsure of how much to worry about symptoms. It can be difficult to discern between what is expected and necessary and what signifies a problem that could be treated or managed better. This challenge highlights the importance of ongoing, patient-specific education and informed reassurance from medical providers and clinical staff.

During times of stress, emotional reactions reverberate throughout the family. For families faced with a new diagnosis of a chronic disease, emotional reactions and accompanying coping strategies vary between family members and across the course of illness. It is not uncommon for the stress of the situation to seep its way into relationships and create division between the patient carrying the diagnosis and his or her family members. Once the permanence of the situation feels real, anger can set in. Family members and caregivers often become targets on which to project feelings of anger, frustration, exhaustion, confusion, and sadness. Furthermore, for some patients, the diagnosis of a chronic health condition can feel isolating in that it sets them apart from others who appear healthy or do not carry the same diagnosis. The same can be true for family members who find their circumstances and routines drastically changed, especially when a chronic disease is diagnosed at a non-normative phase of life.

Depending upon the phase and type of chronic disease, the need for caregiving can span from minimal assistance with medical needs (e.g. going to medical appointments, taking medications, performing at-home treatments) to full-time assistance with activities of daily living (e.g. bathing, dressing, eating). Although fulfilling and necessary in many ways, the demands of long-term, extensive caregiving can lead to emotional and physical exhaustion, relational tension and guilt, and the depletion of financial resources. After a long period of watching a loved one suffer, it is not uncommon for family members to wish for the person's suffering to end, even if that means death. However, these types of feelings are often accompanied by guilt and shame at wishing for this outcome.

A Contextual Perspective on Living with Chronic Disease

As a systemic model of family functioning, contextual therapy is grounded in the concept that a life-changing chronic disease impacts the individual functioning of all members of the family and changes the relationships between individual members. Illness alters personal and professional identities, modifies goals and expected timelines, and adds in often complicated treatment regimens. As challenging and real as these predicaments are, there are also plenty of opportunities for growth for families. With an open mind, priorities can be reset, and expectations can be renegotiated. Connections can be restored within the new reality of chronic illness. Identities can be redesigned in a way that honors both old ways of being and new experiences. Previously unexplored beliefs about health, illness, and the function of the healthcare system become more transparent and able to be discussed.

Caregiving in the context of chronic illness serves many purposes in families and can be viewed through many lenses, all of them true in different circumstances and at different times. Providing care and assistance to one who is suffering from a chronic disease is a challenging, humbling, rewarding, privileging, frustrating, tiring, and worthwhile endeavor. As Jacobs (2006) wrote, "The reality of undertaking sacrifice is that it almost always exacts some toll. The more we choose to ignore that reality, the more the toll is compounded" (p. 84). It is essential to replenish one's personal reserve in order to dig deeper to find the value, despite the cost, of providing care for a loved one with a chronic disease.

From a contextual perspective, caregiving offers opportunities for children, partners, or other loved ones to earn entitlement by giving to someone in need. It may be a way to begin to repay how that person cared for you in another part of life. It may be a way to respond to an intergenerational calling to care for one's aging parents and is part of the family life cycle. It may also feel like a burden to set aside your own dreams and preferences, especially for someone who has caused hurt and pain previously. Regardless, caregiving of some kind (whether completed by the family or a healthcare service) is likely to be needed at some stage of chronic disease. The timelines and level of caregiving needed, of course, are influenced by the rate of progression of symptoms and the level of disability associated with the disease.

Case study 7.1 will be used to describe the story of one family whose journey with type 1 diabetes was complicated by additional life stressors and painful relationships. As in the previous chapter, we will use this story to illustrate how one integrated healthcare team was able to draw from a contextual framework to inform the treatment of this patient and his loved ones. We will highlight ways in which the therapist, medical providers, nursing staff, and community stakeholders collaborated to promote physical and relational healing.

CASE STUDY 7.1

Stevie was 13 when he was diagnosed with type 1 diabetes. He was a black child in a semi-rural, mostly white community, and he lived in a neighborhood where violence and street drug use were frequent and expected. He described drive-by shootings as something he thought about nearly every day. He was raised for the first ten years of life by his mother Shaundra, but he described her as "not really around much." When he was nearly 12, his mom was incarcerated for about a year. He and his three younger sisters—Grace, Tamara, and Jasmine—moved across town to live with their dad Ray, with whom they had never spent much time previously.

Stevie got a mischievous, playful gleam in his eye that he tried to conceal with a straight face when he would harass his sisters; he could frequently be seen rolling his eyes with them, giving them gentle (and sometimes not so gentle) shoves, and cursing at them. As with many young siblings, the girls took on the role of "tattletales" with boldness and felt certain they should report all of his alleged mistakes to whatever adult seemed in charge. They were a rowdy bunch who always seemed to be caught in a scuffle with one another.

About three months after his mom was released from prison, Stevie became very drowsy at school and passed out. When the school nurse became concerned, he was taken to the emergency room at a local hospital. There, he was diagnosed with type 1 diabetes. This was the first time Stevie and his family had ever heard of type 1 diabetes. They were more familiar with type 2 diabetes, which they assumed you got from "eating too much McDonald's." In the emergency room, the treating physician called a diabetes educator to meet with the family and create an initial plan for adjusting diet, checking blood sugar levels, and taking insulin. During this meeting, the family seemed unengaged in the diabetes management conversation and overwhelmed by trying to contain outbursts of sibling rivalry and taking phone calls from extended family members about an unrelated crisis. The diabetes educator felt overwhelmed by trying to continue explaining the importance of type 1 diabetes care in the midst of such a chaotic interaction. She eventually sent them home with some insulin and written instructions, and she encouraged them to make an appointment in the next few days with Stevie's primary care provider. Stevie's mom gave a noncommittal agreement to make an appointment, and the family hurried through the discharge paperwork, eager to leave this hospital.

The hospital hiatus did not last long. In less than a week, Stevie was back in the emergency room with a blood sugar level near 275. He was fatigued, had a headache, and seemed disoriented. This time, his symptoms were so serious that he was admitted to a short stay in the pediatric intensive care unit (PICU) to help stabilize his blood sugar levels and provide additional opportunities for education with him and his parents. Both his mom and dad came to the hospital, but they rarely were in the same room together. Having some difficulty finding a steady job after her incarceration, Stevie's mom worked as a cashier at a fast food restaurant, and his dad worked as a mechanic in a car shop. Never married, their break-up several years ago had been filled with bitter accusations of infidelity and intermittent bouts of physical violence. Now, they barely communicated to plan for their children's care, and the distaste they had for one another was palpable when they were together.

During this PICU stay, the nursing staff insisted that the family spend more time with the diabetes educator, who showed them more extensively how to measure blood sugar levels at home and administer insulin. Although initially disinterested in learning too much, Stevie's parents became slightly more engaged when the PICU staff threatened to call Child Protective Services (CPS) if they did not comply with Stevie's medical recommendations. Although this helped to engage the parents, it made them wary of honestly communicating with the staff about areas of confusion or concern about follow-through with Stevie's care. After a few days in the PICU, Stevie was released back into his parents' care at home.

Less than a week later, he was back in the ER with low blood sugars warranting another stay in the PICU. This pattern continued for several more hospital stays, until Stevie had been in the PICU six times in 2 months. The clinical staff began to place playful bets on whether he would be admitted to their service that day, and they were exasperated that "this family just could not get it together." Some staff were angry that his parents were putting his life in jeopardy. Some were resigned to Stevie's inevitable return and just shrugged it off.

During this time, I (ASH) worked at this hospital as a medical family therapist, and I frequently saw patients and their families in the PICU. During afternoon rounds to discuss patients, I could empathize with the staff members' growing frustration and concern about this boy's health and well-being. I offered to meet with the family to determine underlying factors for poor diabetes management and work with case management to create a plan to support the family in stabilizing their use of socio-economic assistance, their emotions within their relationships, and their management of Stevie's diabetes.

The first time I stepped into Stevie's room in the PICU, I found just him and his mom sitting in the dark. Stevie was entranced in a video game. When I introduced myself and requested a few minutes of their time, he briefly glanced at me and then looked back to his video game. Shaundra, clearly annoyed and tired, raised her voice and told him to "get off that game." Begrudgingly, Stevie put down the game controller but began fiddling with his phone. He made it pretty clear he had no desire to talk or be open. I asked a few questions about how he was feeling that day and what he thought about the doctors and nurses and he provided one- or two-word answers or shrugs. Deciding to switch my focus, I asked if it was OK with him if I asked his mom a few questions. Seeming a bit relieved to be out of the spotlight, he nodded.

After some small talk just getting to know one another, Shaundra finally opened up a bit more. She expressed her stress over having a child with a disease that she did not really understand and seemed to go well or poorly at random. She talked about feeling lonely that her friends were too busy with their chaotic lives to help out, and she was worried about her girls' grades in school, on top of Stevie's illness. Staring at Stevie, she poured out concern that he had been fighting at school and did not seem to get along with anyone, and he just seemed angry all the time. With tears and an end-of-her-wits tone, she said, "I don't know what I'm going to do. If he keeps fighting, he is just going to end up in jail like everyone else. He has got a thick skull, and he just does not seem to get that. He is stubborn like his father." As Shaundra shared this, I watched Stevie's reaction out of the corner of my eye. He was looking away, staring at an opposite wall, trying to show that he was not interested or listening, but I could tell he was tuned in by the changes in his breathing.

I took a few moments to express mutual concern and hope that although this was a difficult time, it also represented a chance for the family to unite over keeping Stevie healthy and adjusting to a new reality: life with diabetes. I inquired about some strengths that Shaundra saw in Stevie. Although she struggled at first to come up with something tangible, she finally admitted that "he is smart—like really smart" and "is really caring when he wants to be." I acknowledged that Stevie's smart and caring nature would be an asset as he learns to manage his diabetes, and I affirmed Shaundra's obvious care for her son and her desire to help him succeed despite a long family lineage of incarceration, dropping out of school, and engaging in family and community violence. I closed up by asking Stevie to show me the video game he was playing, and he seemed much more willing to talk about that. I said goodbye and made plans to return tomorrow for a brief check-in.

When I returned the next day, I found Stevie in his room alone. Shaundra was working, and his sisters were at school. I played video games with Stevie for a bit and then transitioned into asking him, "What do you want to do after high school?" Stevie shared that he loves basketball and wants to play for the Golden State Warriors someday— they were his favorite NBA team. He proudly shared that he helped his own team win every game except one last season, and I asked about how his diabetes had impacted his basketball game. He shared that he finds it annoying to have to stop what he is doing to check his blood sugars and thinks that "insulin is for sissies." Diabetes didn't fit with his idea of a tough basketball player. I helped him draw the connection between needing to be healthy and strong to keep training for the NBA, and that meant eating well and keeping his blood sugars in balance. This connection seemed to make sense for Stevie—he had a reason to care about his diabetes if it meant continuing to play great basketball. Things were going well so far, and I asked about how he thought his mom could help him stay healthy and strong and keep his diabetes in control.

With that question, his face darkened, and he quietly said with a biting edge, "I do not need her help." Realizing I had touched an emotional nerve, I asked him what he meant, and he said, "She is never around. She has her own stuff to deal with. I do not need her." Gently, I reflected his desire to be independent and take care of himself, and he stayed quiet. I tentatively offered, "You know, I might be way off here, but one thing I heard is that your mom was gone for most of last year, and it sounds like you did not get to see her very much. Any chance you learned to take care of yourself so much while she was in jail?" A single tear fell from the corner of Stevie's eye, and he brushed it away hastily. He stayed quiet for a long 60 seconds, and then the emotional tale spilled out.

His mom was put in jail for a violent crime mixed with a drug charge, and he felt abandoned when she was "taken away." She had said she would always be there for him and his sisters, and he perceived her incarceration as a lie that contradicted her promise of stability. He did not believe he fit in with his dad's family with his girlfriend and her children, and he hated that he had to change schools when he moved in with his dad. Nearly everyone in his family had spent at least some time in prison, and he expected he would do the same someday. He acknowledged that part of it was "bad choices," and part of it was "the police having it out for black people." He had no hope that he could avoid jail time or an early death due to violence, and he did not see the point in taking care of his diabetes. Taking care of a chronic disease did not matter when survival and freedom seemed much more difficult to attain.

I thanked Stevie for his openness in sharing his thoughts and his fears with me and stated that I felt honored to be in this struggle with him. I wondered aloud whether his mom might be having the same struggles since life after incarceration can be pretty difficult for many people. He partially acknowledged this with a shrug and an "I guess so." Since he was planning to be discharged from the hospital later that evening, I asked him if maybe I could help him and his mom talk about this some more next time I saw them. He agreed, and I wrapped up the visit for the day.

Unsurprisingly, Stevie was back in the PICU less than a week later with low blood sugar levels. His mom was exasperated because she thought she had been trying to buy healthy snacks and teach him how much insulin to take, but his blood sugar levels did not demonstrate success. Stevie was prone to binge eating candy he bought at school and refused to eat vegetables at home. He preferred chicken and potatoes, and he put up a big fight about not drinking sodas when his sisters had free access to as many sodas as they wanted throughout the week. There seemed to be some tension between Stevie and his mom that day, and I asked Stevie if it would be OK to pick up where we had left off last time we chatted. He begrudgingly nodded, and I provided a brief summary to Shaundra that we had talked briefly about how difficult her absence due to incarceration had been for their family. I described my desire to help them readjust to life together and how that fit with adjusting to life with diabetes; although the details were different in this case, I had had similar conversations with many families in this same hospital. She hesitated before answering, and just said, "It has been hard." I acknowledged that it must be hard to talk about, especially with someone you do not know very well, and she sighed and nodded in agreement.

Throughout the visit, I helped facilitate a conversation between Shaundra and Stevie about their hurts, fears, and resentments related to family reunion and health. Shaundra's primary struggle was with guilt: ending up in jail when she always thought she would be different, feeling ashamed so she refrained from calling her kids more than twice that year, and failing to help Stevie keep his diabetes in check. She was stuck working few hours at a fast food restaurant and brought home burgers for dinner and could barely afford to keep healthy food in the house. She felt deep pangs of guilt for not being able to provide better for her kids. Stevie desperately missed his mom while she was gone but felt unsure about how to react now that she was back, and he held her at an arm's length distance now. He had trouble letting her in and trusting that he could rely on her to help him when he was struggling or feeling down about being the only kid he knew with diabetes.

After hearing Stevie open up about his feelings, Shaundra dropped to her knees beside his hospital bed, and she took Stevie's hands in hers. He looked a bit unnerved but eager to see what came next. With tears streaming down her face, she apologized for leaving him and his sisters alone. She said, "Look, I know I messed up. And I can never take that back. But I need you to know I am so sorry and I want to start fresh today. I am your mom, and you are my only son I have. I do not want to lose you to diabetes or the police or any more bad choices I make. I want us to be close. I want to be there for you. I will do whatever it takes to show you that you can trust me. That is my job—to earn your trust back." The two shared a warm, tearful hug, with sheepish grins back at me after they broke away from the embrace. "What are you staring at?" Stevie said with a bashful look as he wiped away the tears from his eyes.

I wrapped up the session by highlighting the ways in which this family was restoring their connection, starting with that conversation. There was much work left to do with learning about diabetes management, connecting with resources to assist with food security, and forgiving one another and moving past the bitterness and anger of the past. More importantly, there was so much hope present in that day's session. It was a start to forgiveness and creating a new legacy: one of resounding resiliency and rising above the challenges of poverty, violence, and illness.

Conceptualizing the Case

What contextual elements could you begin to identify throughout this case? First, let us conduct an assessment of what we know so far and organize it according to the four dimensions of a contextual framework.

Factually, Stevie was a Black child who grew up in a single-parent home surrounded by instability, violence, and legal troubles. He was the oldest and only male child of several siblings, and he had recently been diagnosed with type 1 diabetes. To his and his parents' knowledge, there was no family history of type 1 diabetes. He was a talented basketball player who had dreams of playing professionally. He enjoyed playing video games. His mom, Shaundra, and his parents worked hard at low-paying jobs, and the family had difficulty in buying food and paying for necessities.

Psychologically, Stevie presented as a child with significant anger and a "tough guy" kind of attitude that kept others at bay. Shaundra expressed guilt over having been an unstable parent due to her own poor choices that ended up in incarceration and lack of emotional availability for her children. Due to the limited nature of therapy in a setting like the PICU, no mental health diagnoses were made, nor were any previous diagnoses identified by the family.

Transactionally, Shaundra's guilt made it difficult for her to lean into re-establishing relationships with her children. Her own woundedness led her to draw inwards instead of risking reaching out. Her children's anger and lack of trust in her incited fear that they would reject her. Her children interpreted her lack of full-hearted engagement with them as more abandonment, which escalated their anger toward her and fueled her reasoning for staying distant.

Concerning *relational ethics*, this family was seriously lacking in trustworthiness and a sense of balance in giving and taking. However, Shaundra's statement of commitment to Stevie in the hospital room showed a move toward restoring a legacy grounded in trust and dependability. She was working diligently to create a new legacy for their family: one of connectedness and mutual love and concern. Her dedication to this new legacy could give Stevie hope in his ability to hold onto the best parts of his family and work toward something beyond the legacy of violence, aggression, anger, and hopelessness.

What to do with all this information as a contextually minded clinician? Only a snippet of this family's story was contained in these few pages, and there are many more curiosities to explore such as:

- What level of loyalty did Stevie feel he was showing to his family by engaging in the same violent behaviors as his many family members who ended up incarcerated?

- What are the most important behaviors for Shaundra to engage in that would show Stevie that she is making a sincere effort to earn back his trust?

- What legacy would Shaundra's family like to write for themselves as the story of how they bounced back from disconnection and violence?

- What steps would be involved in helping Ray and Shaundra co-parent their family and provide their children with stability? How might this improve their children's relationships with both of them?

Planning Interventions

Once you understand more about the context of this family's source of guilt, lack of trustworthiness, and misguided loyalty, you can build a plan for additional interventions. Change began to occur in the hospital room when Stevie risked being open with his mom about his hesitation to trust her to help with his diabetes. Shaundra presented Stevie with a sincere apology and rededicated herself to being a mom and helping care for him. In this family, it seems essential to address all aspects of time: past, present, and future.

For a child who has learned to guard himself from a parent in the past, it can be difficult to re-establish trust, even when a parent has apologized and seems sincerely motivated to change. Maio, Thomas, Fincham, and Carnelley (2008) found that forgiveness between an adolescent and a parent has the potential to spill over into creating a more positive family environment beyond just the parent-child subsystem. With a clinician's help, Stevie could determine what kind of forgiveness he wished to extend to his mom. Hargrave (2001) described contextual-based forgiveness as including various "stations," beginning with gaining enough insight to stop the hurt from reoccurring. At the heart of the second stage of forgiveness is understanding the context of why a loved, trusted person hurt you. Although it doesn't take away the pain, understanding the background and the reasons why a painful thing happened give another meaning to the story, one that doesn't solely involve a personal attack. The third and fourth stations must be paced appropriately, and they include giving the opportunity for rebuilding trust and offering overt forgiveness as part of restoring the relationship.

In Stevie's case, his mom wished to be different and not end up falling into legal troubles. When she did repeat this family pattern, her guilt kept her even more imprisoned, telling her that reaching out to her children would be even more harmful to them. Thus, she stayed at bay, and Stevie felt more isolated and alone. Although that is the extent of what was shared in this case study, a clinician working with this family could help thicken the story by asking some additional questions such as:

- To Shaundra: "From your childhood, can you relate to some of the feelings Stevie has expressed, like feeling confused why someone he loved did not reach out to him and feeling alone when he needed some help?"
- To Stevie: "How does the pain of your mom not reaching out to you compare to a time when a friend hurt you and was not very good to you?"

The goals of these types of questions are two-fold: (1) to help Stevie learn the context by which his mother left him feeling abandoned, isolated, and uncared for and (2) to help Shaundra remain in a place where she can compassionately respond to her son's hurt without letting her own defensive guilt take over.

With a present focus, the therapist could assist Stevie in describing some instances in which his mom shows behaviors that increase his trust in and connection with her. This type of intervention would help Stevie begin to reevaluate the current status of his relationship with his mom and identify specific instances in which she shows she is working to earn his trust. This method—restoring trust in another person by re-evaluating present circumstances rather than offering someone a blank slate and pretending harm has not been done—can feel much safer for those who have been victimized. In addition, it continues to show Shaundra that she is accountable for her actions, not just her words, in showing her son her dedication to earn his trust. Although Shaundra, like many parents, may feel entitled to earn this back quickly, the therapist may need to remind her that forgiveness is a process that knows no certain timeline. Likewise, the process of restoring relationships is more topsy-turvy than many expect, and forgiveness and patience are likely to be necessary on both sides.

Of note, a key intervention with this family included collaboration with case management and diabetes education from a registered nurse. Although repairing the relationship between Stevie and his mom was essential in building a support system, it would have been short-sighted to assume that this automatically would lead to improved diabetes management. Rather, practical skills and additional resources were needed. The case management and diabetes education teams in the hospital taught the family how to choose cost-effective, diabetes-friendly snacks and meals that Stevie was likely to eat and that fit with the family's very limited income. This took several tries to find the right balance and get Stevie on board with choosing less carbohydrate-heavy snacks. Eventually, his visits to the PICU dwindled, and his less frequent low blood sugar episodes could be managed more swiftly in the emergency department without a multi-day stay in the PICU. It is likely that this was due to improved food choices and reduced relational stress in Stevie's life, since research supports the connection between high stress levels and destabilization of blood glucose levels (DeVries, Snoek, & Heine, 2004). Both Stevie and Shaundra reported feeling quite pleased with their ability to prevent most problems with too high or too low levels of blood sugar.

This serves as a good reminder that basic needs such as food, shelter, and safety are essential to address before higher-level constructs such as relational healing can really become the center of focus. With additional resources to add financial buffering to provide healthy foods for the family, Shaundra was able to devote additional time, patience, and energy to supporting Stevie in his management of stress and diabetes. Finally, future-focused interventions could focus on helping Stevie and his mom work together to create a vision of their family's continued healing. As with all families with a member with a chronic health condition, they have an important, difficult task ahead: how will they define their family's relationship with diabetes, and how will they use their relationship and combined skills and resources to manage diabetes? Thinking of their story, one positive way to reframe this journey with diabetes is that it has presented the family with an opportunity to address past barriers to trust, loyalty to a common cause, and fairness. Diabetes offered a common problem for Shaundra and Stevie to bond together and face. One question for this family might include, "Now that your diabetes is more stable, what will keep you connected and working together?" Another key item to assess is how Stevie would like his mom to continue being involved in his diabetes management as he grows older, more responsible, and more capable of caring for himself.

Key Learning Points

In summary, this case provided an excellent example of how underlying tensions and a culture of poverty interacted to prevent one teenage boy from effectively managing his diabetes. It also described the necessity of a team-based approach, with diabetes educators and medical providers to give tips on disease management and a therapist to address complex family dynamics that added stress and prevented appropriate coping strategies. With a chronic disease made more difficult by family dynamics, it is essential to address past, present, and future components of time in order to heal old wounds and plan for preventing future problems.

REFERENCES

Chasens, E. R. & Luyster, F. S. (2016). Effects of sleep disturbances on quality of life, diabetes self-care behavior, and patient-reported outcomes. *Diabetes Spectrum, 29*(1), 20–23.

DeVries, J., Snoek, F., & Heine, R. (2004). Persistent poor glycemic control in adult type 1 diabetes: A closer look at the problem. *Diabetic Medicine, 21,* 1263–1268.

Hargrave, T. (2001). *Forgiving the devil: Coming to terms with damaged relationships.* Phoenix, AZ: Zeig, Tucker, & Theisen.

Holt, R. G., de Groot, M., & Golden, S. H. (2014). Diabetes and depression. *Current Diabetes Reports, 14*(6), 491–493.

Jacobs, B. J. (2006). *The emotional survival guide for caregivers: Looking after yourself and your family while helping an aging parent.* New York, NY: Guilford.

Maio, G. R., Thomas, G., Fincham, F. D., & Carnelley, K. (2008). Unraveling the role of forgiveness in family relationships. *Journal of Personality and Social Psychology, 94,* 307–319.

Renn, B. N., Feliciano, L., & Segal, D. L. (2011). The bidirectional relationship of depression and diabetes: A systematic review. *Clinical Psychology Review, 31*(8), 1239–1246.

Rolland, J. S. (1994). *Families, illness, and disability: An integrative treatment model.* New York, NY: Basic Books.

Rolland, J. S. (1997). A journey with hope, fear, and loss: Young couples and cancer (pp. 139–150). In S. H. McDaniel, J. Hepworth, & W. J. Doherty (Eds.), *The shared experience of illness.* New York, NY: Basic Books.

Smith, K. J., Béland, M., Clyde, M., Gariépy, G., Pagé, V., Badawi, G., . . . Schmitz, N. (2013). Association of diabetes with anxiety: A systematic review and meta-analysis. *Journal of Psychosomatic Research, 74*(2), 89–99.

Tomm, K. (1998). Interventive interviewing: Part III. Intending to ask lineal, circular, strategic, or reflexive questions? *Family Process, 27*(1), 1–15.

Turner, J. & Kelly, B. (2000). Emotional dimensions of chronic disease. *Western Journal of Medicine, 172*(2), 124–128.

World Health Organization (2017). Noncommunicable diseases. Retrieved April 27, 2017 from www.who.int/topics/noncommunicable_diseases/en/

Chapter 8

Tangled Minds

Contextual Perspectives on Mental Health

Whereas the previous two chapters focused on acute and chronic health concerns that were primarily related to physical health, this chapter will focus on challenges in promoting health with those with comorbid mental health disorders. Since depression, anxiety, and substance use disorders represent some of the most common mental health conditions present in both traditional mental health and medical settings, these conditions will be the main focus of the chapter. To frame the discussion, we will present a case study of treatment for a middle-aged woman with major depressive disorder and intractable migraine headaches and her husband who struggled with alcohol abuse.

SYSTEMIC PERSPECTIVES ON MENTAL HEALTH CONDITIONS

According to the 2001–2003 National Comorbidity Survey Replication, 34 million American adults, or 17 percent of the adult population, reported comorbid medical and mental health conditions during a 12-month period (Alegria, Jackson, Kessler, & Takeuchi 2003; Druss & Walker, 2011). With a shortage of trained mental health professionals and slow-to-change stigma surrounding mental health conditions, primary care is often an entry point for people to seek treatment for mental health symptoms (e.g. depression, anxiety, poor sleep) that coincide with physiological symptoms and disease processes. Primary care often becomes a de facto mental health service center for many patients, especially in rural or more remote areas that lack a mental health workforce (Kessler & Stafford, 2008). Many patients first discuss concerns and worrisome symptoms with their primary care provider before seeking psychotherapy and the services a mental health clinician can provide.

There is evidence to support the use of psychotropic medication such as antidepressants to treat mental health disorders like depression. However, the effectiveness of these pharmacologic treatments depends on a variety of factors, including the severity of symptoms, patients' pharmacogenetic profile, and adherence to treatment recommendations (Institute for Quality and Efficiency in Healthcare, 2017). As systemic clinicians, we believe that psychotropic medications alone are not enough to create lasting change in behavioral patterns, coping strategies, or relationship problems that lead to distress for patients.

Rather, mental health symptoms such as depression and anxiety are inevitably entangled with individuals' relational histories and current experiences with others. It is important to note that both medical and mental health issues can lead to what one patient of mine (ASH) called "tangled minds" (uncertainty, confusion, fear, worry) and "tangled relationships" (ones that seem to cause rather than relieve pain). Health-related issues, whether physical or mental in nature, have a way of exacting a toll on individuals, as well as their relationships with friends, family, and co-workers. Therefore, we propose that asking about the association between mental health symptoms and personal relationships should always be part of a comprehensive assessment in both medical and mental health treatment setting. Understanding more about relationships helps clinicians illuminate triggers for symptoms as well as resources and strengths to capitalize upon during treatment.

Systemic Views of Depression

From a systemic perspective, depression is far more than an imbalance in serotonin levels or an individual problem that is the leading cause of disability in U.S. adults between the ages of 15 and 44 (Anxiety and Depression Association of America, 2016). Recent research (e.g. Brady, Kangas, & McGill, 2016) continues to highlight the importance of educating families about the many nuances of depression symptoms and addressing family-level variables. Let us return to the four dimensions of assessing human experience using a contextual lens to compile a systemic, multifaceted view of depression.

Factually speaking, there are studies that suggest complex associations between factors such as age of onset, early life events, temperament, family history of depression, and gene identification and an individual's experience of major depression (e.g. Docherty et al., 2017; Keller et al., 2017; Kendler & Aggen, 2017). On a psychological level, higher levels of cognitive distortions—such as all-or-nothing thinking, catastrophizing, externalizing self-worth, perfectionism, and should statements—are associated with higher levels of depression symptoms (Blake, Dobson, Sheptycki, & Drapeau, 2016). Furthermore, interactions between family members are uniquely intertwined with depression symptoms. Depression symptoms impair family members' responses as parents (Thomas, O'Brien, Clarke., Liu, & Chronis-Tuscano, 2015; Wilson & Durbin, 2010) and romantic partners (Whitton et al., 2007). A systematic review conducted by Santini, Koyanagi, Tyrovolas, Mason, and Haro (2015) reported that individuals who described having relationships with others where they perceived strong emotional and instrumental support in large, diverse social support networks were less likely to report depressive symptoms, calling attention to the ways in which social interactions can also serve as a protective factor from depression.

From a contextual point of view, depression is inevitably intertwined with people's sense of self and relationships with others, and there is sufficient evidence to support the use of systemic treatments to address this episodic disorder (Carr, 2014). As we have described in previous chapters, violations of love, trust, and loyalty in individuals' lives can have a profound effect on the way that they view the world and their expectations of interactions with others. Without protective social factors and personal resiliency, repeated experiences of poorly balanced relationships and painful experiences can lead to feelings of hopelessness, helplessness, and worthlessness that can present as depressive symptoms.

Systemic Views of Anxiety

Often comorbid with depressive disorders, anxiety disorders comprise the most common mental health disorders experienced by Americans

(Kessler, Chiu, Demler, & Walters, 2005; Kroenke, Spitzer, Williams, & Löwe, 2009). In fact, an estimated 40 million U.S. adults, roughly 18 percent of the population, meet criteria for an anxiety disorder (National Alliance on Mental Illness, 2017). Anxiety symptoms include both emotional (e.g. feelings of worry and dread, feeling tense and jumpy, restlessness and irritability, acute awareness of signs of danger) and physical elements (e.g. pounding or racing heart, sweating, tremors, fatigue, sleep problems, gastrointestinal distress). Not surprisingly, these symptoms can have a profound impact on the ability to function within relationships.

From a contextual perspective, there are a variety of potential triggers for anxiety disorders—some of which are related to facts and psychological states, and some of which are relationally created and maintained. As with depression, there is evidence to support the role of genetic (e.g. Sotnikov et al., 2014) and life experiences such as trauma (e.g. Kuo, Goldin, Werner, Heimberg, & Gross, 2011) that predispose individuals to experience anxiety symptoms, as well as thought patterns that lead to poor emotional regulation and heighten anxiety symptoms (e.g. Carthy, Horesh, Apter, & Gross, 2010; Hertel & Brozovich, 2010).

There are various systemic theories that describe ways in which anxiety is influenced by and influences family systems. Attachment theory, foundational in emotionally focused therapy, proposes that insecure attachments fuel relationship distress and conflict (Johnson, 2004), where partners or family members are deeply worried about whether their loved ones will meet their emotional needs and respond in a way that seeks to build intimacy and connection. These emotional fears and the chronic conflict or distance that accompany them often present as individual anxiety symptoms. In another example, Priest (2015) used Bowen family systems theory to frame research findings that individuals who had been exposed to family abuse and violence were more likely to report symptoms of generalized anxiety disorders (GAD) and romantic relationship conflict. In that study, individual differentiation—an ability to remain emotionally present with others while also reacting autonomously—helped to mediate the effects of family abuse and violence on GAD symptoms.

Chronic conflict or distance within relationships is likely to fuel individuals' anxiety symptoms and inhibit their ability to engage in treatment, unless properly addressed by treating healthcare providers.

As with depression, there is evidence to support the use of systemic and relationally oriented therapies to treat anxiety disorders. Carr (2014) noted that couple and family-based therapies are most effective for three specific types of anxiety disorders: agoraphobia with panic disorder, obsessive compulsive disorder (OCD), and post-traumatic stress disorder (PTSD). Carr wrote, "Systemic interventions create a context within which families can support recovery, and a forum within which family interaction patterns and belief systems that often inadvertently maintain anxiety disorders can be transformed" (p. 174).

Systemic Views of Substance Use Disorders

Substances misused and abused can vary greatly, but general themes found in addiction—secrecy, denial, shame—are fundamental processes involved in the maintenance of the disease. Depending upon the substance, acute or chronic episodes of misuse can lead to serious health issues, legal troubles, financial problems, and even fatality for the individuals who engage in risky, unhealthy substance use. In addition to the impact of addiction on physical and financial health, the internal impact on one's emotions and self-worth can be just as devastating and helps to perpetuate a self-sabotaging cycle.

Beyond the individual impact of substance use disorders, there are myriad ways in which families, friends, and others in the community are affected by substance misuse, too. For example, Haverfield and Thiess (2016) described the various types of stigma that adult children of parents with alcoholism face and explored the ways in which family communication patterns changed, depending upon the gender of the adult children and the severity of the parent's alcoholism. One important take-away from this study's findings was the suggestion that increased opportunity within the family to talk openly about the parent's alcohol problem was associated with adult children having a clearer understanding of their parent's illness and their role in the family. Thus, one goal of systemic intervention to support families affected by substance misuse should be facilitating open, honest communication to express concerns and understand what the family is experiencing.

As systems thinking reminds us, the relationship between families and substance misuse, of course, is not unidirectional. Rather, there are also tangible ways in which family patterns and interactions increase the likelihood of risky substance use and threaten recovery. As summarized by Hawkins, Catalano, and Miller (1992), poor parenting practices, high conflict within the family, a low degree of bonding between parents and children, and parents and older siblings' modeling of inappropriate substance use have been shown to increase the risk of adolescent and later life substance use disorders.

Although a variety of different therapy approaches have been applied to treatment of substance abuse, a growing body of research has high-lighted the value of addressing substance issues systemically (e.g. Carr, 2014; O'Farrell & Clements, 2012; Steinglass, 2009). Timing family involvement in treatment may matter. For example, Edwards and Steinglass (1995) determined that there is a significant benefit in involving family members in motivating persons struggling with alcohol use disorders to enter treatment, but the benefits of involving them throughout treatment are only marginally higher than individually focused treatment. Another study by Morgan, Crane, Moore, and Eggett (2013) even found that the average cost of family therapy to treat substance use disorders ($124.55) was lower than that of individual therapy sessions ($170.22) due to a decreased number of average treatment sessions needed (2.41 for family, 3.38 for individual). Family therapy sessions also offered a lower recidivism rate (8.9 percent) compared to individual therapy sessions (12 percent). Other studies have suggested that the timing of involving families in treatment matters. Thus, there is a compelling case to provide systemic interventions to treat issues like substance use disorders, which have undoubtedly systemic consequences and prevention strategies.

CONTEXTUAL VIEW OF MENTAL HEALTH CONDITIONS

Although it can be difficult to generalize across mental health conditions due to the immense variation in individual experience and symptom type and severity, there are a few ways to consider how contextual concepts such as loyalty, family legacy, and justice apply to individuals' experiences with mental health disorders. When using a contextual framework for working with individuals and families affected by mental health disorders, a few key ideas come to mind.

When individuals are diagnosed with a mental health condition such as depression, they must work over time to develop a legacy of how this label, for better or worse, fits into their lives and shapes their experiences. They must become gatekeepers, determining how and when they allow their depression symptoms to shape their experiences and what they wish to maintain control of, despite the presence of depression. This same process applies to families who support an individual with chronic mental health difficulties. Legacy building is a relational process as much as it is an individual one.

Similarly, families must determine how loyalty fits into the picture as they support a loved one with a diagnosed mental health condition. The central question to be answered is, "How much does the family perceive this as one person's problem versus a problem they must face together?" Loyalty means making difficult choices between what *I* want as an individual and what *the family as a whole* needs. At times, loyalty to the family's well-being may mean individual sacrifices and choosing to forego a desire for the greater good of the family. A mother may choose to take time off work to help her adult son make it to a psychiatry appointment that he is worried about, or a brother may choose to call his sister more often when he knows her depression symptoms are on the rise. However, if all members in the family have a goal of maintaining loyalty to the family system, the result will be a balance that sustains love, care, and trustworthiness over time. As one can imagine, loyalty struggles become more intense and difficult in families where trust has already been broken, imbalance in giving and receiving has gone unchecked, and feelings of resentment prevail.

Expectations of how much the balance shifts must be crafted around various dimensions of a person's life. We think the four dimensions of a contextual therapy framework provide a useful starting point. *Factually,* it is important to consider the diagnosis and symptoms included, treatments being pursued and available for future consideration, and severity of distress and functioning. How the person makes *psychological* meaning of the diagnosis and its impact on his or her life is an essential component that influences ideas about what sort of support and assistance is needed (from minor to very substantial). The current status of *interactions* with family members, friends, neighbors, and other community members is also an important factor in determining if the balance should be shifted from time to time to accommodate greater need for care and support during phases of increased and decreased struggle.

Many mental health conditions have an episodic nature, with periods of remission and relatively good functioning and flares which bring greater distress and relatively poor functioning. Thus, the nature of relational ethics—the balance of giving and taking over time—must account for these episodes, and expectations should shift accordingly. There will be times when greater support is needed from family and friends, as well as times when this is not necessarily desired as much. Open, honest conversations within support systems are essential to ensure expectations are clear and can be matched to the current situation.

To illustrate these contextual concepts and how they can apply to the treatment of a patient with comorbid medical and mental health problems, we will next present a case study. This will be followed by a conceptualization of the case and some sample interventions that were or could have been included.

CASE STUDY 8.1

Donna, a 44-year-old Latina female, presented to her primary care physician (PCP) to establish care as a new patient. She had been diagnosed years ago with a rare form of muscular dystrophy that involved weakness in her limbs and ptosis, or droopiness in her eyelids. Although the disease has a progressive nature, the only symptom she reported at this early stage was significant fatigue. "I just feel so tired all the time," she explained. She reported feeling as if she wanted to sleep all day and had trouble motivating herself to get out of bed, go to her part-time job as a caregiving aide for her neighbor, and complete household tasks. Donna also described severe migraine headaches four to five days per week that severely impacted her mood and ability to be productive at work and at home. She provided a long list of medical treatments she and previous physicians had tried, with little relief. She reported she had recently seen a neurologist who thought Botox injections were her "last option" but that her muscular dystrophy prevented that from being a viable option for her.

After gathering some additional information related to Donna's health history, her PCP suggested to her that there may be a chance she was also suffering from depression. He asked his staff to administer the Patient Health Questionnaire (PHQ-9; Kroenke, Spitzer, & Williams, 2001), and Donna scored a 24 out of a total of 27 points, signifying severe depression symptoms. Donna endorsed symptoms of depression including anhedonia, hopelessness, fatigue, poor appetite, low self-esteem, and trouble concentrating. Most concerning, she had marked that she thought about wanting to kill herself more than half the days of the last two weeks. When her PCP started a conversation with her about her responses on the questionnaire, she said, "I have felt this way for a long time. I just do not know what to do about it."

Fortunately for Donna, her primary care team included me (ASH) as an onsite integrated behavioral health provider. Donna's PCP shared with me his concern for Donna's depression symptoms, and he believed there was a strong bidirectional relationship between her frequent migraines and her depression. Together, we hypothesized that severe headaches without treatment providing significant or lasting relief put her at greater risk for increased depression symptoms, and her depression heightened her awareness of and susceptibility to experiencing pain. Donna and her PCP had already discussed initiating an anti-depressant medication, and she was open to talking to a behavioral health provider. The PCP and I set a goal for my initial visit with Donna to focus on (1) assessing the nature and severity of her suicidal ideation and creating a plan for safety and (2) formulating a treatment plan aiming to reduce her depression symptoms and teach her additional skills for managing her migraines.

When I entered the exam room after Donna finished meeting with her PCP, the room was dark and only lit by a single lamp. I pointed to it and said, "Just a guess . . . it probably doesn't help your migraine when all the overhead lights are on?" Donna smiled weakly and shook her head. I explained my role as one of her PCP's colleagues and described my background as a medical family therapist. I summarized what I understood of her depression, migraines, and muscular dystrophy from her PCP and asked what else she felt was important for me to know about her health. She described unintentional weight loss of 15 pounds in the last three months and difficulty falling asleep at night; her thoughts about her family and limited income kept her awake until the early morning. She described her headaches as feeling like a pounding or squeezing and made worse by light and loud sounds. She said, "When my head hurts, all I want to do is lay down and sleep. Or throw up. It's a toss-up."

I empathized with the difficulty of exhaustion and ongoing pain and then asked about her support system. Donna hesitated. "My family is alright," she stated cautiously. I asked her to tell me more about them, and she sighed. She described that she had been married to her second husband for 19 years, and they had one daughter who was now married and pregnant with her first child. I inquired about how her troubles with migraines and ongoing fatigue have impacted her relationship with them, and she described feeling guilty since she could not do as much for her daughter as she would like.

Her husband, she said, was a different story. She described his tendency to "drink more than he should," and she estimated he drank six to eight beers most days of the week. She reported that when he was relatively sober, he was unengaged and standoffish but generally kind. She described him as "a mean drunk" when he started drinking, though she denied any physical violence occurring between them. His aggression took the form of harsh words and ignoring her less subtly than he did when he was sober. When I asked how alcohol had impacted her marriage, she said, "You know, I know he cannot really help it, and I feel like I should do more to help him. For years, I have tried to keep him afloat and make sure he does not lose too many jobs or start too many fights with people. But I am tired, just so tired. I can barely take care of myself these days, and I do not know how I can keep up with him, too."

My concern for Donna's suicidal thoughts came to the surface, and I informed her that her PCP had shared with me her responses to the questionnaire she had just completed. I said that I wanted to ask more about her response to the last question, and her eyes immediately welled up with tears. She began rubbing her temples and said, "I think about it a lot, you know? Life just seems so hard these days, and I do not want to do it anymore. It just doesn't seem worth it." I affirmed my understanding that she had been suffering quite a bit and asked how she had thought about giving herself some relief from that suffering. She described having thoughts about killing herself, mostly confined to fantasies about driving her car off a cliff near her home. She had these thoughts nearly every day, but she reported them being relatively easy to remove from her active mind, except when they were highest at a level of a 7 out of 10.

When I asked her why she had not acted on these thoughts, she said, "I always think of how much my family needs me. What would happen to my husband and my daughter if I were gone? Plus, I know I would go to hell if I killed myself. God would not like that." Her religious beliefs and her intense loyalty to her family prevented her from engaging in behavior that would harm herself, but it was not enough to keep the thoughts entirely at bay. Donna said, "I know I haven't yet, but I'm just afraid someday I will be so depressed I will not be able to stop myself." She reported her suicidal thoughts as being at a level 2 out of 10 that day, with no active plan to act on the thoughts. She thought talking about it helped reduce the loneliness of not wanting to live like this. I described for her my goal of helping her come up with a plan to reduce those thoughts and keep herself safe next time she found them on her mind again.

Together, Donna and I came up with a plan that tapped into her strengths of family loyalty and connection with God. When she noticed these thoughts, she would call her daughter to chat and distract herself from the thoughts leading her to feel hopeless. She described not wanting to be a burden on her daughter and not wanting to worry her about the suicidal thoughts, so she wanted to keep the conversation lighter. She thought her daughter would respond well and want to talk with her more often. She listed a few people to call as back-up options in case her daughter was busy, and she set a plan to read through some of her favorite comforting Bible verses to ease her distraught mind as well. She had an app with the Bible on her phone, so even if she was driving and started experiencing these suicidal thoughts, she could pull over and read a few verses until she was calmer.

Armed with these strategies, a new medication, and information for the crisis phone line and how to reach our clinic's on-call physicians after-hours, Donna and I said our goodbyes and planned to check in during her next primary care visit in a month. When I saw Donna next, she described no change in her headache frequency or severity. She was, however, feeling some benefits of the antidepressant medication with reduced feelings of hopelessness, although she still felt physically tired much of the time. She described a cycle in which she would push herself to accomplish a great deal on the days when she was feeling well and then pay for it the next day with rebound headaches and debilitating exhaustion. We discussed the importance of pacing in order not to perpetuate that cycle, and she decided to set a timer on her phone to remind herself to take a short break to relax every hour on the days when she was feeling good and had much to get done.

I asked her how else I could be helpful. She stated she wanted to continue to work on her depression symptoms. The most troublesome symptom for her these days was her perception of her own existence as worthless. She described that she was unable to work as many hours as she would like due to her headaches (and her depression, she now realized), which meant her husband was the primary financial provider. She felt guilty about putting this strain on him, and she thought this might be responsible for his drinking to excess. Money was tight, and they fought about it a lot. I validated Donna's sincere care for her husband and wanting to support him as a partner, and I provided some psychoeducation on the disease process of addiction, which I suspected her husband suffered from, according to her reports. This helped untangle her fatigue and depression symptoms from being a direct cause of his drinking behaviors, and slowly she began to hold herself less directly responsible for his drinking. She was able to see her own illnesses as part of the context, not the immediate precursor, for his drinking behaviors.

My hunch was that Donna was giving to the relationship with her husband much more than she gave herself credit for. I shared this hunch with Donna, and she looked at me blankly. "Maybe," she offered slowly. I brought out a piece of paper and said, "I would like to test out if that might be the case. Do you mind if I write a few things down and we take this step by step?" She nodded. Knowing it was easier for her to delineate what she thought her husband provided for her, I asked her to begin listing a few things her husband did for her.

The trickier part was helping Donna see what she herself contributed to the family. At first, she deflected with an attempt at humor and said, "I just try to stay out of everybody's way, but I am still a drain. I just try to keep myself a drain in the corner." I redirected her back to the question, and she began to actually give it some thought. "Well," she said, "I am usually the one who does the grocery shopping, even when I do not feel so well. I know money is really tight, so I try to buy whatever is on sale or use a coupon." I affirmed her resourcefulness in making smart grocery

Table 8.1 Ledger

Giving	Receiving
Donna grocery shops with good financial judgment and savvy money-saving skills	Husband works full time to provide income and insurance benefits for the family
Donna tries to remain positive with her health and not complain too much to family	Husband spends time with their daughter and her husband
Donna cleans up around the house	Husband grills dinner about once per week
Donna makes dinner most nights of the week	Husband occasionally fixes broken appliances and fixtures around the house

store decisions and working with limited funds, and I encouraged her to keep going with her list (see Table 8.1). She described trying not to complain too much about her headaches and tiredness, cleaning up around the house when she had a good day with a little more energy, and making dinner most nights of the week.

Upon looking at this list, Donna seemed surprised. "I guess I do more than I think," she admitted. She was also able to express some gratitude for what her husband did to contribute to the family, but she had a wistful look on her face. I asked her if there was something she wished might be in that receiving column that wasn't really there right now. She hesitated for a moment and said, "My husband is good to our daughter and he is good at helping around the house when he is not too drunk, but I feel like our marriage is pretty empty. We never talk like we used to, and we do not really spend any time together that is not working on a project." I inquired if this was something she thought might help alleviate some of her burden of coping with her health problems and her depression symptoms, and she nodded emphatically.

Donna seemed hesitant to invite her husband to join for any sessions to discuss ways to rebuild intimacy and connection in their marriage within the context of her poor health and his drinking behaviors. Respecting her wishes, we continued with individual therapy sessions for several more visits, focusing on various aspects of how to find the balance between (1) caring for her family and taking pride in being able to contribute something to them and (2) setting boundaries in determining what was appropriate, based upon what she received from others, the type of the relationship (parent-child vs. spouse), and her health and well-being. Within several sessions, Donna reported feeling more in control of her ability to choose how much to try to take care of others vs. how much to expect and ask for from others. This improvement helped lift some of the physical burden of trying to do too much for others, resentment and self-worthlessness that fueled her depression, and hopelessness about having any kind of quality of life while coping with chronic depression and frequent migraines.

Conceptualizing the Case

What contextual elements could you identify in Donna's story? First, let us assess what we know so far and organize it according to the four contextual dimensions.

Factually, Donna is a Latina female in her forties who has been diagnosed with a rare form of muscular dystrophy and migraine headaches. Her daily functioning is most impacted by feeling chronically fatigued and in significant pain. She has been married twice, and her second husband (by her report) engages in risky alcohol use. She has an adult daughter who lives in the same town who is expecting her first child.

Psychologically, Donna's motivation to complete any tasks has severely dropped off as her physical symptoms have worsened. She engages in a significant amount of negative self-talk, telling herself things like, "You do not deserve to have anyone take care of you" and "You just need to be more selfless for now; eventually someone will change and treat you better." Her depression leads her to feel sad, worthless, and hopeless. She is tired—physically, spiritually, and emotionally.

Transactionally, Donna gets stuck in a pattern where she feels distraught that her husband does not provide her with enough emotional support and intimacy to withstand the turbulence of poor health. Her depression kicks in and her negative self-worth messages become louder, and she then feels guilty for not taking better care of him so she denies her own emotional needs and tries to focus on just being there for him. Although this serves to diffuse any potential conflict in the short term in their relationship, it perpetuates long-term feelings of loneliness and isolation. Moreover, it fails to provide Donna with the love and care she is entitled to ask for and receive as part of this intimate relationship.

It also prevents her husband from accepting responsibility and accountability for contributing emotional care to his partner.

Concerning *relational ethics*, Donna vacillates between perceiving her relationship as being imbalanced in the direction of her receiving too much or too little. Either way, it feels unsatisfying because she has chosen loyalty to her relationship (by way of "not rocking the boat") at the expense of her own well-being. However, this long-standing pattern has tarnished the nature of trust she has in her relationship to fulfill her needs and provide her with strength, comfort, and care during her own times of weakness and pain. This lack of trust in this relationship is likely also to feed into her hesitation to reach out to her own daughter, either because she fears her daughter will let her down by not providing emotional support or she will place an unfair expectation on her daughter to meet her emotional needs.

Although the written description serves to organize what we initially know about Donna and her complicated relationship with health and her family, additional curiosities that could help shape further intervention include:

- How could Donna redefine loyalty to her family in a way that does not come at the expense of prolonged self-sacrifice that exacerbates her physical and mental health problems?
- How have Donna's difficulties in determining a reasonable balance of giving and receiving been influenced by her experiences in childhood and in her family of origin? What models of relationships within her family can she identify that appeared more well balanced? Poorly balanced?
- Given Donna's husband's drinking problems, how could she balance (1) asking for additional assistance and care from him to support her own health journey and (2) providing him with ongoing support in his journey to reduce risky drinking behaviors?

Planning Interventions

The assessment I conducted with Donna's PCP revealed some key focus areas to address with the goal of alleviating depression symptoms and giving her some additional perspective on her frequent migraines and how to cope with them. With a link between her depression and her physical stress and pain symptoms (headaches), one key area of focus became how to help Donna reduce her loneliness and hopelessness related to her family relationships. By improving the quality of her relationships and enhancing her own self-worth, her treatment team was hopeful her depression could lift and help alleviate the ways in which her body responded in a physical way to emotional pain.

Several sessions in, I asked Donna what she felt would help rebalance her relationship with her husband and make it one that offered her a more fulfilling experience. She thought about this question for a moment and said, "I think I need to speak my mind more." Over the last few weeks, Donna realized she had been stifling herself from asking him to engage with her more, to help her, to show care and concern for her. She had realized that it was not fair to expect him to change if she did not tell him how she felt and what she wanted. She decided to make a goal of talking to him about this in the next week when he seemed relatively sober. She realized alcohol got in the way of her doing this as consistently as she would like, but she was not ready to ask him to quit drinking and she did not think he was ready to give it up either.

The next week, Donna reported that she had to explain several times to her husband why these demonstrations of care were important to her, but they had had the conversation. She described it as feeling "a bit awkward at first," but she had asked him to try these two things to show her he cared for her: (1) make coffee for her in the morning and (2) ask her how her day was each evening and actually listen to the answer. She described his attempts to do these things over the last week, and she realized she would need much more over time to rebuild balance in their relationship. But, she said, this was a start. She needed to know he cared about her well-being and he knew how something like a simple cup of coffee showed her that he was willing to do a task that meant something to her. She described that she felt more able to give herself permission to ask for additional assistance or kindness on the days when she felt poorly and had a migraine.

Another area of intervention included drawing some more distinct boundaries between what she could ask to receive from her family and what she wished to keep giving to others. Donna recognized that she had been letting so many things slide over the years that she had a difficult time not feeling guilty for not doing enough, even when it was coupled with resentment over doing too much while getting little in return. I asked Donna to think about what she would use to gauge what she felt comfortable in continuing to give while accounting for her need and desire to receive love and care, too. How would she know when she needed to speak up to realign the balance? Donna came up with this internal checklist of questions she'd use as a way to make decisions on a case-by-case basis.

- Do I feel stressed or angry? Do I feel sad? Why? Do I feel like I can safely share these feelings with this person?

- If I were to do this task for this other person, how would that help them in the short term? How do I see this playing out in the long term?

- Will this cost me anything I am not willing to give up?

- What would I look for in the future to see this balance restored? How can I ask for that if it is not initiated by someone else?

Over time, Donna used this internal checklist in a variety of ways to better understand why she would feel torn between feeling unworthy to receive more from others and also angry they didn't show enough love and care to her. Her depression symptoms became more manageable, and she felt more hopeful about her ability to continue growing and coping, which led to less frequent and less intense thoughts about suicide. Although she continued to experience migraines on a fairly frequent basis, she continued to work with her PCP on medical management and felt she could give herself permission to be gentler with herself instead of trying to shame herself into better health.

Key Learning Points

With the complex interactions between body and mind, it is intuitive to recognize that mental health and physical health symptoms often become tangled together. Even with today's medical advances and technology improvements, it can be difficult to discern how much a headache is caused by biological susceptibility or psychosocial stress. However, this speaks to the importance of medical and mental health providers addressing presenting complaints of patients with a holistic view that looks at how people's bodies process physiological, psychological, and relational stress and how to help patients work toward creating meaningful, satisfying relationships. Although we recognize that relationships can be the source of significant stress and heartache, we also strive to recognize the ways in which balance can slowly be restored and relational resources such as trust and loyalty can be harnessed for the good of the identified patient and his or her family and community.

REFERENCES

Alegria, M., Jackson, J. S., Kessler, R. C., Takeuchi, D. (2003). *National comorbidity survey replication* (NCS-R), 2001–2003. Ann Arbor: Inter-University Consortium for Political and Social Research.

Anxiety and Depression Association of America (2016). *Understand the facts: Depression.* Retrieved February 25, 2018 from https://adaa.org/understanding-anxiety/depression

Blake, E., Dobson, K. S., Sheptycki, A. R., & Drapeau, M. (2016). The relationship between depression severity and cognitive errors. *American Journal of Psychotherapy, 70*(2), 203–221.

Brady, P., Kangas, M., & McGill, K. (2016). "Family matters": A systematic review of the evidence for family psychoeducation for major depressive disorder. *Journal of Marital and Family Therapy, 43*(2), 245–263.

Carr, A. (2014). The evidence-base for couple therapy, family therapy, and systemic interventions for adult-focused problems. *Journal of Family Therapy, 36*(2), 158–194.

Carthy, T., Horesh, N., Apter, A., & Gross, J. J. (2010). Patterns of emotional reactivity and regulation in children with anxiety disorders. *Journal of Psychopathology and Behavioral Assessment, 32*, 23–36.

Docherty, A. R., Edwards, A. C., Yang, F., Peterson, R. E., Sawyers, C., Adkins, D. E., . . . Kendler, K. S. (2017). Age of onset and family history as indicators of polygenic risk for major depression. *Depression and Anxiety, 34*(5), 446–452.

Druss, B. G. & Walker, E. R. (2011). Mental disorders and medical comorbidity. *The Synthesis Project. Research Synthesis Report, 21*, 1–26.

Edwards, M. E. & Steinglass, P. (1995). Family therapy treatment outcomes for alcoholism. *Journal of Marital and Family Therapy, 21*(4), 475.

Haverfield, M. C. & Theiss, J. A. (2016). Parent's alcoholism severity and family topic avoidance about alcohol as predictors of perceived stigma among adult children of alcoholics: Implications for emotional and psychological resilience. *Health Communication, 31*(5), 606–616.

Hawkins, J. D., Catalano, R. F., & Miller, J. Y. (1992). Risk and protective factors for alcohol and other drug problems in adolescence and early adulthood: implications for substance abuse prevention. *Psychological Bulletin, 112*(1), 64–105.

Hertel, P. T. & Brozovich, F. (2010). Cognitive habits and memory distortions in anxiety and depression. *Current Directions in Psychological Science, 19*(3), 155–160.

Institute for Quality and Efficiency in Healthcare. (2017). Depression: How effective are antidepressants? Retrieved February 25, 2018 from www.ncbi. nlm.nih.gov/pubmedhealth/PMH0087089/

Johnson, S. (2004). *The practice of emotionally focused couple therapy: Creating connection* (2nd ed.). New York, NY: Routledge.

Keller, J., Gomez, R., Williams, G., Lembke, A., Lazzeroni, L., Murphy, G. M., & Schatzberg, A. F. (2017). HPA axis in major depression: Cortisol, clinical symptomatology, and genetic variation predict cognition. *Molecular Psychiatry, 22*(4), 527–536.

Kendler, K. S. & Aggen, S. H. (2017). Symptoms of major depression: Their stability, familiarity, and prediction by genetic, temperamental, and childhood environment risk factors. *Depression and Anxiety, 34*, 171–177.

Kessler R. C., Chiu, W. T., Demler, O., & Walters, E. E. (2005). Prevalence, severity, and comorbidity of twelve-month DSM-IV disorders in the National Comorbidity Survey Replication (NCS-R). *Archives of General Psychiatry, 62*(6), 617–627.

Kessler, R. C. & Stafford, D. (2008). Primary care is the de facto mental health system. In *Collaborative Case Studies in Integrated Medicine: Evidence in Practice* (pp. 9–21). New York, NY: Springer.

Kroenke, K., Spitzer, R. L., & Williams, J. B. (2001). The PHQ-9: Validity of a brief depression severity measure. *Journal of General Internal Medicine, 16*(9), 606–613.

Kroenke, K., Spitzer, R. L., Williams, J. B. W., & Löwe, B. (2009). An ultra-brief screening scale for anxiety and depression: The PHQ-4. *Psychosomatics, 50*(6), 613–621.

Kuo, J. R., Goldin, P. R., Werner, K., Heimberg, R. G., & Gross, J. J. (2011). Childhood trauma and current psychological functioning in adults with social anxiety disorder. *Journal of Anxiety Disorders, 25*(4), 467–473.

Morgan, T. B., Crane, D. R., Moore, A. M., & Eggett, D. L. (2013). The cost of treating substance use disorders: individual versus family therapy. *Journal of Family Therapy, 35*(1), 2–23.

National Alliance on Mental Illness (2017). *Anxiety Disorders.* Retrieved February 25, 2018 from www.nami.org/Learn-More/Mental-Health-Conditions/Anxiety-Disorders

O'Farrell, T. J. & Clements, K. (2012). Review of outcome research on marital and family therapy in treatment for alcoholism. *Journal of Marital and Family Therapy, 38*(1), 122–144.

Priest, J. B. (2015). A Bowen family systems model of generalized anxiety disorder and romantic relationship distress. *Journal of Marital and Family Therapy, 41*(3), 340–353.

Santini, Z. I., Koyanagi, A., Tyrovolas, S., Mason, C., & Haro, J. M. (2015). The association between social relationships and depression: A systematic review. *Journal of Affective Disorders, 175*, 53–65.

Sotnikov, S. V., Markt, P. O., Malik, V., Chekmareva, N. Y., Naik, R. R., Sah, A., . . . Landgraf, R. (2014). Bidirectional rescue of extreme genetic predispositions to anxiety: Impact of CRH receptor 1 as epigenetic plasticity gene in the amygdala. *Translational Psychiatry, 4*(e359).

Steinglass, P. (2009). Systemic-motivational therapy for substance abuse disorders: an integrative model. *Journal of Family Therapy, 31*(2), 155–174.

Thomas, S. R., O'Brien, K. A., Clarke, T. L., Liu, Y., & Chronis-Tuscano, A. (2015). Maternal depression history moderates parenting response to compliant and noncompliant behaviors of children with ADHD. *Journal of Abnormal Child Development, 43*(7), 1257–1269.

Whitton, S. W., Olmos-Gallo, P. A., Stanley, S. M., Prado, L. M., Kline, G. H., St. Peters, M., & Markman, H. J. (2007). Depressive symptoms in early marriage: Predictions from relationship confidence and negative marital interaction. *Journal of Family Psychology, 21*(2), 297–306.

Wilson, S. & Durbin, C. E. (2010). Effects of paternal depression on fathers' parenting behaviors: A meta-analytic review. *Clinical Psychology Review, 30*(2), 167–180.

Chapter 9

Seeking Healing at the End of Life

This chapter will focus on ways to help families prepare for the death of a loved one and to help aging individuals heal injustices experienced throughout their lifetime. When we become aware of death drawing near, conversations often shift to talk about things like what legacy this person will leave behind, how that fits within the greater family story, and how this death will influence multiple generations of family members. There are many factors—age, amount of time between time of diagnosis and death, connections within the medical community, and more—that dramatically shape patients' and families' experiences of preparing for the end of life. To illustrate some of these differences, we will present two case studies: (1) a patient diagnosed with amyotrophic lateral sclerosis (ALS) and his process of strengthening his bond with his wife before his death and (2) a patient diagnosed with an aggressive form of cancer and her process of fighting for more time with her husband and young children.

ALL IN THE FAMILY

As an inevitable fact of life, death is a certain experience all humans share. Some die at a young age, and some die at an old age. Some spend a long time waiting for death to arrive, and some are caught by surprise when death comes. Some die alone, and some die surrounded by caring medical teams and loved ones. Although aging brings an often sad, frustrating, painful awareness of mortality and the nearness of death, Hargrave (1992) pointed out that the experience of aging and preparing for the end of life is not solely a negative one. Rather, "in the midst of the pain and the fear and the sadness, life gives the family one of the last great opportunities to resolve old issues and empower one another with love and trust" (Hargrave, 1992, p. 3) Aging provides a strengthening exercise beyond physical fitness; it has the power to strengthen family ties. What does it mean to let life give the opportunity to empower a family to choose love and trust over resentment and injustice? We'll explore just that question in this chapter.

In families with balanced relational ethics, members of the older generation who are preparing for the end of life feel empowered and invited to pass on wisdom they have gained through life experience and relationships to members of younger generations (Hargrave, 1992). Through sharing their life stories and experiences, they shape the fabric of the family and promote shared values and belief systems. These stories captured in a life review set a foundation for the family's value-driven legacy: how to face adversity, how to represent yourself to others, what to expect from family members, and more. However, when lack of trust and injustice have prevailed in a family, this "passing on" of wisdom becomes stilted. Wise words become lost in a sea of painful emotions like anger, resentment, and fear. Moreover, defense mechanisms like denial and justification can be used to cover up the injustices that have occurred in families. The task of contextually minded clinicians is to courageously and compassionately bring these to light so the injustice can be corrected, not swept under the rug once more.

Hargrave (1992) poignantly used the metaphor of a wound to describe the inevitable hurts that occur in families over time and influence their process of preparing for the end of life of a loved one. When members of multiple generations live alongside one another for decades, there are bound to be bumps and bruises. Fortunately, most of these minor hurts heal relatively easily with time and appropriate care. However, there are some wounds that cut so deeply into the flesh of a family that they leave permanent damage and scars. When this occurs, smaller wounds continue to make the pain worse. Remedy after remedy may be tried, but it may seem that nothing eases the pain. "Like the body in major illness," Hargrave wrote, "relational survival is in question"

(p. 145). Individual members may grow distant from one another, and forgiveness seems like a long-lost idea. This type of family trauma often seeps into individuals' interactions with others, calling into question the trustworthiness and justice in any relationship, personal or medical. If these relational wounds are left untreated and continue to fester, it makes dealing with the physical experience of death that much more painful, both for the person preparing for death and those connected to him or her.

The rise of hospice and palliative care has led to a recognition of the need to help families seek a form of healing that goes beyond physical cure. When a family remains open to the possibility, the dying process of a loved one can lead to intimate conversations about what really matters: family, shared past, and unknown future (Byock, 1997). As Byock reflected on his experience working with families involved in hospice care, "Dying from a progressive illness had provided them with opportunities to resolve and complete their relationships and to get their affairs in order" (p. 31). The process of dying well does not need to be rushed or feared. Rather, it means that individuals show courage in accomplishing tasks that are meaningful to them and their families and continue to grow throughout the process. Teams supportive of a dying process like this— meant to be engaged with instead of feared— give themselves and their patients the opportunity to expand the possibilities of relational healing and growth, restoring love, care, trust, and balance.

Next, we will share two clinical cases that highlight two unique patient cases and how families approached the end of life in a way that promoted healing and restoration of relationships.

CASE STUDY 9.1

Years ago, I (ASH) worked as a medical family therapist in a neuromuscular clinic designed to meet the needs of patients with amyotrophic lateral sclerosis (ALS), also known as Lou Gehrig's disease, and their families. If you aren't familiar with this progressive disease, ALS is a neurodegenerative condition that affects nerve cells in the brain and spinal cord. With the death of motor neurons, patients gradually lose the ability to perform voluntary movements like speaking, eating, moving, and breathing. Although there is a hereditary component to one form of ALS, between 90 to 95 percent of cases are not linked to a family history and are considered sporadic (ALS Association, 2017). Unfortunately, there is not yet a cure for this disease, although there are a variety of treatments to help manage symptoms and slow the progression of the disease in some cases.

This clinic that operated out of a general neuromuscular clinic one day each week was specifically designed to meet the variety of needs introduced by ALS. A multidisciplinary staff consisted of neurologists, a social worker, a physical therapist, nurses, a respiratory therapist, a durable medical equipment specialist, and a medical family therapist. During new patient consult and follow-up appointments, each patient had the chance to visit with a number of these team members to address concerns and make proactive plans to improve their quality of life and adjustment to this disease.

Dr. Jones, one of the neurologists in the practice, asked me to meet with Joe and his wife Betty. He was concerned that Joe was experiencing some depression, and he could sense growing tension between the husband and wife. He worried that Betty was experiencing some caregiver fatigue, as was common with so many other families seen in this clinic. I agreed to step in and visit with Joe and Betty at the end of their appointment that day.

Having been diagnosed with ALS nearly a year ago, Joe was a delicate, fragile-appearing man in his seventies. Betty, his wife of over fifty years, faithfully attended every appointment. She had clearly taken on the role of speaking for Joe—figuratively and literally. Although they had some assistance from home health, Dr. Jones mentioned that she was Joe's primary caregiver at home and preferred to do as much as she could herself. My first impressions of her were that she was fiercely protective and exhausted in a way that sleep could not fully remedy.

ALS follows a different symptom progression for every patient, and I began by asking a few questions about how the disease had most impacted Joe's life so far. He had first noticed weakness in his legs and arms a little over a year ago, and he was now confined to a wheelchair, barely able to use his arms. His speech had also begun to slur over the last few months, which made it difficult for him to communicate with others. He reported that previously he had an active social life and would visit with friends several times a week, but he now preferred to spend several hours each day playing computer games. Joe's voice betrayed his sadness, despite kindly saying, "That's just how it goes, I guess. It's alright." Glancing out of the corner of my eye, I noticed that Betty coldly stared out the window and slowly shook her head.

I paused and asked how I could be helpful for the two of them today. Betty looked at me without speaking for a moment, seeming like she was deciding whether to let me into their world. She pursed her lips and said, "Well, my husband is dying. And all he wants to do is play on the computer. I'm so damn sick of it." She described a couple of stories in which she wanted to go out and "live life while they have it," and all Joe wanted to do was sit in a dark office at home on the computer. I listened carefully and validated her pain at losing her beloved husband and her intense desire to be close to him. Betty looked surprised, and her face visibly softened. "Yeah. That is what I want."

I began to understand that Betty's anger and resentment had deep, deep roots in sadness and fear of loss, and I wanted to expose those roots rather than focus on the anger so clearly at the surface. I realized that, in order for our interactions to be successful, I had to understand her anger and frustration and help her speak from a place of more authentic, primary emotion so her husband could hear her. Building my relationship with Betty, I explicitly told her how much I valued her being here today. Beyond being a source of medical history or an anxious caregiver for the patient, I viewed her as essential and equal in importance to helping their family manage life with ALS. I noticed a visible change in her openness to talk after saying this.

I asked Betty if she would be willing to try something with me. She looked at me skeptically, but she agreed. I said, "I think your husband needs to hear something straight from you. You just told me how you are missing him already, and you are scared of losing him. You want to spend time with him. But can you turn to him and tell him more? I think he needs to hear this. This is too important to hear secondhand from me." She sighed quietly, and then she turned to him. She told him, "I know it seems like I am always mad lately. And I am sorry about that. I just get so frustrated. I thought we were going to have so many more years together, and it feels like we have been robbed of that time. I want to make the most of what we have, and right now, I just feel like a nurse or maid taking care of you. I just do not understand why you want to sit in that dark room all the time." She felt abandoned before death had even taken her husband. Joe looked at me, seeming a little bewildered, and I motioned to him to respond to her.

"Well," he started slowly and deliberately, "It is just easier, I guess. I am embarrassed for people to see me this way. Nobody wants a guy who talks slow and can hardly walk." I watched as Betty teared up, and she said, "I do. I want that guy. I do not want to go through this feeling like I am alone when you are still here." During the rest of the conversation, she was able to come to see that his reliance on playing on the computer by himself was not intended to be an avoidance of her but a way to protect himself from the shame he felt about his deteriorating physical condition. This shift in perspective made a huge difference that it was something they could grieve over together and strategize what to do about it.

I framed the issue as one in which what Joe might want for himself is peace and quiet by himself, but their marriage needed something else. We talked about other times in their marriage when they had had to choose to put aside what they individually wanted so they could be loyal to their relationship and support one another. Together, Joe and Betty started brainstorming a few ideas on how they could spend some time together in ways that met Betty's deep desire for connection and Joe's desire for some privacy from the outside world. We said our goodbyes, and I planned to see them in two months at their next appointment.

At that next visit, Dr. Jones told me that Joe's speech and movement issues were about the same, with only minor changes noticed. However, the energy in the room felt noticeably different when I entered. The two were sitting on the same side of the room, quietly chatting, and Joe smiled in a genuine way. I asked how things had been going at home since we had last talked, and they both reported things were going much better. Betty described that she felt loved and appreciated by the way Joe had talked to her during the last appointment, and she had been pleasantly surprised by her husband's active efforts to spend more time with her over the last few weeks. Their love was blossoming in simple, beautiful ways. They sat on their patio to drink coffee each morning, and they played cards each afternoon.

Realizing that they did well with one-on-one facilitated conversations, I asked Betty to turn to her husband and tell him what it meant to her that he had made these changes. Taking his hands in hers, she said, "It shows me you are still here, and you love me. I can trust you to be here when I need you. It gives me the strength to do all the things I just have to do to try and keep you healthy." Joe smiled and patted her hand, and he said, "You mean everything to me. I don't know how I would do this without you. I like spending time with you, even when I don't feel comfortable being so exposed with other people and wondering what they are thinking about the old sick guy." Over the last two months, they had worked hard to restore their connection and solidify that as the foundation for them to face adversity and painful circumstances.

I asked them what impact they thought their renewed connection might have on the rest of their family. Betty said she noticed she felt less of a need to call and complain to their daughters, and she thought they appreciated this. She knew she did not want to place a burden on them, and she thought they had a more positive relationship as a result of her feeling better about her connection with her husband. Joe said he felt a little more confident about going out in public a couple of times because if he knew Betty was on his side and loved him despite his sickness, he did not really care what everyone else thought. I highlighted the lessons they were sharing with their children and grandchildren, showing the possibility of love and connection despite preparing for death and how they leaned into the challenge as opposed to shying away from it. "What a legacy you are creating, one simple day at a time," I said. They smiled, seeming quite proud of themselves, and we made plans to follow up in another two months.

I saw Joe and Betty twice more, and each time, our conversations were filled with tears, laughter, and tender looks. At our last meeting, Joe's speech had declined so that he primarily communicated through painstakingly writing on a notepad. Sensing that he was nearing the end of life, I asked him what he felt was unfinished in his life. He wrote that he still needed to keep showing his wife how much he loved and appreciated her. I asked him how he might show her how deeply he cared for her, and he wrote, "By getting rid of this ALS." I felt the pain associated with these words in my own heart, and I glanced at Betty, whose eyes quickly filled with tears.

I observed out loud that it seemed to me like the weight and reality of this incurable illness had sunken in, and Betty nodded quietly. Joe wrote, "I know I cannot make it go away. Want to but cannot." Betty mentioned how difficult it was for them lately since they wanted to hold and kiss each other, but the stiffness in Joe's arms and paralysis in his facial muscles made this near impossible. With their restored emotional closeness, they yearned for physical closeness, too.

I suggested to them that even though ALS was interfering with Joe's ability to speak his words of love to his wife and hold her in his arms, they could still experience deep intimacy through gazing into each other's eyes and by holding each other's hands in their own.

Before I even finished speaking this suggestion, Joe startled me by quickly struggling to sit up in his wheelchair and turning the chair to face his wife. This took a great deal of effort for him, and I was surprised by this sudden movement. I had the feeling that I was meant to simply watch the moment taking place in front of me, so I sat quietly. He turned to his beautiful wife of 53 years, and he reached eagerly for her hands. She seemed surprised, too, but eagerly awaited what came next. He looked deeply into her eyes, and he slowly pulled her hands to his mouth. Her eyes filled with tears as he said to her with unmistakable words: "I love you." It was as if he simply could not bear to wait until later to tell her this. Betty wept fresh tears and clutched her husband close, and I felt incredibly honored to witness these tender moments, all in an exam room in a busy clinic on a Monday morning.

Joe died at home less than a month later, and I called Betty a couple of weeks later to check in. She reported feeling a mixture of emotions—relieved that her husband was no longer suffering yet filled with sadness that he was no longer on this earth. She planned to move to Vermont to be closer to her oldest daughter's family. She expressed gratitude for the time they had shared together at the end and that she was so thankful she had so many happy memories of their quiet times together during Joe's last few months. She said, "It is enough to keep me going for the time I have left here, knowing how hard he worked to love me."

Conceptualizing the Case

When I first met with Joe and Betty, they were individually grappling with the weight of a disease like ALS. They were hurting and feeling desperately alone, isolated on separate islands of grief. Joe felt the weight of a poorly understood and greatly feared disease that left him unable to function on his own, and his self-consciousness about his body's decay prevented him from recognizing the beauty of the relationship he could have with his wife. Betty's stress from serving caregiver duties without the reward of an intimate emotional connection left her with anger and resentment, which kept Joe at bay and made her feel unapproachable and bristly. Their individual pain led to additional heartache in their relationship.

By engaging in difficult conversations about the struggles they faced individually and what they needed from their spouse, they redefined their marriage as a safe haven instead of another source of pain. From a contextual perspective, they rebalanced the relationship. Despite Joe's inability to provide physical assistance in the home, he was able to provide his wife with tender, loving care and appreciation, which was incredibly valuable currency to her. I suspect that Joe and Betty had built a deep reserve of trust and balance in their long-lasting marriage, which is why the damage was relatively quickly repaired once they had someone help facilitate conversations.

Planning Interventions

For Joe and Betty, key interventions were housed in meaningful conversations where they were encouraged to talk directly to one another, instead of through a clinician. A key change moment occurred early in the process when Betty was able to express the roots of her frustration (a lack of energy-restoring time with her husband in exchange for caregiving labor) in a way that showed emotion softer than anger. Another key element was facilitating Joe's openness to hearing Betty's frustration and sharing with her why he was hesitant to leave the house and resorted to time alone on the computer. Hearing each other's individual thought processes and concerns helped clarify that the separation between them wasn't intended to be punishment or abandonment. Redefining the reason why they had drifted apart gave them a common goal to work toward instead of fighting each other, building loyalty to a shared cause and to each other.

In preparing for Joe's death, the concept of legacy came up after the couple started making progress. In our experience, it seems that conversations about legacy creation work best when a family has made some progress, and it can be a useful way to highlight specific changes and capture a value that the family holds dear. Plus, it reminds the family members present for the therapeutic work that their actions impact more than just themselves and have the power to shift culture throughout the rest of the family system. In this case, Joe and Betty talked about their desire to create a legacy that showed their younger family members that sickness can actually bring a family closer together and give them opportunities to show love more freely and openly. To help facilitate legacy-focused conversations, clinicians can ask questions like:

- "What story do you think it tells about your family that you have lived alongside this disease in this way? How close is that to the story you want it to be?"
- "What impact do you think this time of preparing for ___'s death will have on your grandchildren?"

Key Learning Points

Though this couple endured physical and emotional suffering through-out the course of ALS, Joe and Betty represent an excellent example of a couple who changed their story at the end of Joe's life. Rather than drifting apart and getting lost in resentment and unspoken burdens, they had the courage to share their needs and fears with each other. Instead of facing these difficulties alone, they faced them together. This restored connection helped give Joe the courage to face death and Betty the courage to face life as a widow, knowing their relationship with each other was secure had emboldened them. Though I did not have the chance to speak with any of their other family members, Joe and Betty's growth will likely ripple into the rest of their family, weaving a story that personal growth and relational intimacy does not end with a life-changing, life-threatening diagnosis.

CASE STUDY 9.2

When I (ASH) was working in a family medicine residency clinic, I was asked to join a conversation between two residents and a faculty member. They were describing how they each had come to know her in different ways over the last week. Jana, a young woman in her late thirties, had come to the clinic for the first time about two weeks ago, complaining of general fatigue and acute episodes of lower back pain. She had been in a wheelchair for about twenty years after she was in an accident while horseback riding during her teenage years. Aside from several miscarriages and a stillbirth, she had been relatively healthy for most of her life. Her new primary care doctor did a physical exam and ordered some labs to be drawn, but the etiology of the pain and fatigue wasn't clear. They made plans to follow up as needed.

Several days later, the clinic was notified that Jana was in the emergency room. The back pain had intensified in severity, and she reported significant nausea, weakness, and fatigue. This time, a second resident cared for her during his rotation working in the ER. Along with the ER physicians, he decided to order some imaging and additional labs, which showed signs of cancer. They couldn't tell what specific type of cancer yet, but they broke the news to Jana and her husband Tim. The couple was in shock, and they could hardly find the words to ask questions. They quietly went home and scheduled a follow-up appointment with Jana's PCP for two days later.

It was during this follow-up appointment that I was asked to meet with Jana and Tim and help them make sense of this confusing, obscure cancer diagnosis. When I walked in the room, I could feel the heaviness. Tim gave me a weak smile, but Jana mostly sat slumped in her wheelchair looking at the floor. Before diving in to discuss the cancer diagnosis, I asked a few questions about the town in which they lived, their children, and life in general. Tim worked on the family's farm, where their primary crop was corn, and they lived on property adjacent to Jana's parents. They described living close to family as a major help during busy planting and harvesting seasons since they could help watch their two young children.

After they seemed more comfortable, I said, "As part of the team here, your doctors let me know that they've given you some news that was probably pretty difficult to hear. Can you tell me more about what you took away from what they've told you so far?" Tim looked down at the floor, and Jana said quietly, "Well, I've got cancer. And nobody knows what it is yet, but they're working on it. Once we know that, then we can start treatment." I affirmed that this seemed to be in alignment with what I understood of her case, too. I asked her about what went through her mind when she heard the word cancer, and she paused.

"Well, I thought to myself, Jana, you have survived a fall from a horse. And you have survived the death of one of your babies and a bunch of other tragedies. So either you did something to make God really mad, or you can survive this, too." I reflected back that part of her felt like she was being punished with this terrible diagnosis, and the other part of her wanted to believe she is strong enough to withstand the treatment and continue living for her family.

Jana went on to describe a strong will to live that focused on being able to see her babies grow up and continue taking care of her husband and her aging parents. With deep sadness in her voice, she said, "I am not ready to give up yet. I have got too much left to do." I then turned to Tim and asked for his thoughts at this early stage of cancer diagnosis, and he just shrugged. He simply said, "I am here. We will get through this. That's all I can really say." We wrapped up the conversation at today's visit, and I closed by explaining how I typically help families who are wrestling with unclear diagnoses and serious illness. I described that I would continue working with their physician team and provided them with some contact information to get in touch with me if they needed to before their next scheduled appointment.

I saw Jana at her next appointment with her primary care provider about two weeks later; there was still no major news about her diagnosis. Her pain was significant at times in her lower back, abdomen, and pelvis, but overall, she was functioning fairly well. She said she was trying just to enjoy watching her children play. We discussed some of Jana and Tim's discomfort with not having a full diagnosis and treatment plan, but they understood that her doctors could not plan a reasonable course of treatment without knowing what type of cancer had infiltrated her body. The hospital lab would call in a few days with the full pathology report, and they were hopeful they could move forward then.

One week later, I received a message in the electronic health record that Jana had been admitted to the hospital for severe pain and fatigue. The pathology report from the local hospital was inconclusive, and the complexity of the cancer required further workup from a nationally recognized specialty lab. Her treating physician had requested that I meet with them for continuity of care and provide any support needed. This physician mentioned privately to me, "It is not looking good. Scans show the cancer is advancing, and I would not give her a good prognosis. Unfortunately, we cannot really treat it properly until we figure out more answers, so we are still in a holding pattern. Whatever this is, though, it is aggressive." She mentioned that she had tried to tell the family that information, but her words were met with resistance and disbelief. Jana and her parents desperately wanted to believe an answer would arrive and a cure would save her. As I often do in these situations, I wrestled with how to balance a dose of reality in the situation with the need for hope and restoration. I decided to see how the family was doing, and I made plans to visit the next day.

When I walked into the hospital room the next day, Jana was sleeping, but her husband motioned for me to step outside with him. Tim and I found a quiet, private room just down the hall to meet in, and he gave me a wistful, wry smile and said, "I just did not know who else to talk to. I feel like I am going crazy here." I nodded and said, "Hospitals tend to have that effect. What is on your mind today?" He sighed, and tears came to his eyes as he said, "It has been weeks. We still don't have a name for this cancer, and we don't know what it is. How are we supposed to fight it if we don't even know what it is? This is crazy." I reflected back the stress this must be placing on them to be facing such an uncertain, unnamed enemy and that the waiting for answers is often one of the hardest parts of illness. I noted that oftentimes this stress is not just confined to hospital stays and wondered aloud if it had found its way into their home life. With a heavy sigh, he said, "This is harvesting season, and we are supposed to be moving house soon. I should be out in the fields working or taking care of the kids at home, but I just cannot leave Jana. She needs me here, even if I can't do anything to help her." That last sentence struck a chord with me, and I asked him to tell me more about that feeling of helplessness.

Tim was quiet for a minute, then tears streamed down his face. He recounted how he and Jana met, and even though she was in a wheelchair even then, he knew she had a powerful spirit within her. He was immediately attracted to her strength and fortitude. They thought they might never be able to have children, and despite the grief they experienced through miscarriage and stillbirth, they were now raising three healthy children together. "But," Tim said, "I can't do it all alone. I never let myself think this until now, but I think there's a chance she really might not make it. The doctor says time is just passing as we are waiting for answers, and I can't do a damn thing to help my wife. She's suffering, being taken over by some cancer, and all I can do is sit by and watch her wither away. She hurts, and I can't do anything for her. What kind of husband does that make me?"

I was quiet for a moment, and I said, "Tim, I hear so much pain in your voice. This is torturous. But I am not so sure that the torture of this situation means you can't do anything for her. Sure, you might not be able to run that pathology report for her. You might not be able to cure her cancer. You might not be able to take away all her physical pain or her fear. But you can do something for her and for your children. You are not as helpless as the darkness would have you think." Tim was silent for some time and then nodded. He said this reminded him of when they lost their child in a stillbirth and Jana fell into a deep depression for several months. He shared how it took him a while, but he learned how to be with his wife and comfort her during that time; he realized that he could not take away the pain of losing a child, but she needed him to step up and be there for their other child and just to surround her with love and patience and pray with her. I asked if he thought he could do something similar here. He wiped his eyes and nodded. "Yeah, I can be with her. That is what I signed up for, right? I am not going anywhere." We briefly talked over a few ideas of how he could "do something" for her, and he was able to name a couple of tasks to provide both emotional and physical support to his hurting wife.

Two days later, I made another visit to see Jana and Tim, but just Jana was in the room at this time. She said she was feeling pretty tired but could talk for a few minutes. She held her stomach, and I could tell she was in pain. "Pretty pathetic, huh?" she said with a small, self-deprecating laugh. I shared that I thought it took a lot of courage to withstand that level of pain, and she playfully rolled her eyes. "Yeah, that is what Tim says too." Before I had a chance to get any words out, Jana said, "Look, I am glad you talked to Tim. I think he really needed that. He has been so worried about me, and I am trying not to worry too much over here. I know what Dr. Dane said, and I know it is serious. But I just can't give up. We still are waiting on answers from that other lab, and I am going to hold on for better news. My babies need me. I'm not ready to let go. There is too much left to do."

I shared with Jana that I was impressed with her powerful will to live and how committed she was to be a good, loving, courageous mother to her children. I said, "I will be honest, I did not go to medical school, and I do not know about the medicine side of cancer treatment nearly as much as your doctors do. All I know is what they have told me, and it sounds similar to what they said to you. I think a lot of us are frustrated with not having the answers we want right now, so I understand your desire to hang on to a hopeful, good outcome as long as you possibly can. Right now, we are not ready to talk about what the end could be like. I sense that."

Jana nodded, and I noticed her eyelids starting to grow heavy. The pain medication must be settling in, I thought. "But I was thinking, one question I will leave you with is: what lessons do you want to make sure you share with your kids from the last few weeks? That is something you can work on, even from the hospital, and enlist the help of your husband and your parents. Because in the end, regardless of how long you are here on this earth, teaching your kids how to make sense of the good and the bad in life, that is what really matters." Jana nodded again, clearly growing more sleepy, and I said my goodbyes. As I quietly shut the door to her room and waved hello to her nurse down the hall, I remember wishing that we had more time to talk but accepting that she needed her rest. We can pick up where we left off next time, I thought to myself.

The next time did not come as I had planned. Jana was discharged soon after I saw her, and she had gone home to wait until we received further word from the pathology lab. About a week later in the family practice clinic, one of the resident physicians who had worked on Jana's case came to me, looking tearful. "Jana's gone." I was stunned. "Gone? As in she died? How?" I asked. Joined by one of the attending physicians, the resident sat down and told me what she had learned from piecing together notes sent over from a smaller local hospital in a town about an hour away from our clinic. From what we could tell, one of the family members had found Jana unconscious in her bed at home, and they had called an ambulance to take her to the nearest hospital. The doctors there did all they could to revive Jana, but she died shortly after arriving at the hospital.

We sat there quietly, reflecting on how quickly the time had passed and how few answers had been provided in what led Jana to perish so quickly. Tears were shed, hugs were shared, and condolence cards and phone calls were planned. Slowly, we gathered ourselves up and prepared to see other patients. This was a relatively rare experience for me as a therapist to have a patient die so suddenly. Many physicians, however, become accustomed to what Ofri (2013) called a "daily dose of death," although their emotions are also quietly tucked away from public view (p. 98). In this busy medical clinic, death seemed to drift away as quickly as it had come, and the next patient became the focus.

Conceptualizing the Case

I worked with Jana and her family for a short period of time, so I learned only a sliver about the context of their lives. However, the content I gathered and the processes I observed in and between family interactions gave me some insight into how to apply a contextual framework in interactions with this family.

Factually, Jana was a young wife, mother, and daughter. She suffered from a very aggressive form of cancer that quickly brought harm to her body and impacted her functioning. She had already experienced significant interaction with the medical system due to other health events, including a fall off a horse that led to her use of a wheelchair, several miscarriages, and a stillborn child.

Since I did not work with the children or the couple's parents in this situation, I learned most about Jana and Tim's *individual psychologies.* In his desperation watching his wife suffer, Tim attached a meaning of "I am a bad husband if I cannot save my wife" to this experience. Although I suspect this was something he continued to grapple with for some time, we were able to alter this meaning by allowing him the space to see ways in which he could be a loving, attentive husband even while his wife was dying and he could not stop that fact. Jana's desperation came from her much shorter than expected life, as well as her anxiety over dying and leaving her children without a mother. Her words led me to think she thought she would be abandoning her husband and her children if she died while they were so young. Although I didn't have interaction with the family in the week leading up to her death, I cannot help but wonder whether this continued to be her thought until the end or if she reached a place where she could prepare herself mentally and emotionally for the inevitability of death and the possibilities it would bring to the family even in the midst of great sadness.

Transactionally, I believe both Tim and Jana were each trying to show the other how strong they were: Jana by fighting off the cancer and going into remission and Tim by keeping his wife alive and the cancer at bay. In some ways, this helped draw them together as they fought against a common enemy. If I had had more time to interact with this family, I would have inquired about how they were able to balance their shows of strength and willpower and a softer, more intimate connection that allowed them to be vulnerable and transparent with each other about their fears and their grief.

Relational ethics was something that Jana and Tim had built over time. During our one-on-one conversation, I got the sense that Tim slowly came to realize that his bond with his wife hinged on his willingness to be trustworthy and caring, not to save her from death. He recognized the value of caregiving, the sacrificing of his time to work in the fields to be physically present and loving. Although they had a history of learning this during previous tragedies, Tim's loyalty to his wife during her experience with cancer wove another thread of sacrifice and commitment to one another in their family legacy.

Planning Interventions

Because my time working with this family was short, interventions were fairly limited. When I spoke with Jana during that final hospital stay, my closing question to her ("What lessons do you want to teach your children through this experience?") was meant to do two things: (1) refocus on intergenerational longevity that extends beyond a single human life and (2) affirm to Jana that I thought she still had value for her family, despite her body's revolt against health. This is something I have found immensely important over the years when working with patients crippled by disease and disheartened by a lack of independence and physical strength. My steadfast belief in their ability to contribute to their families and communities, regardless of physical ability, is a cornerstone of my work within a contextual framework and reminds patients of their enduring value.

During my conversation with Tim, my words were relatively few, but I chose them carefully. I gently nudged him in the direction of realizing the strength of his role as a husband hinged on more than just physical tasks and items to be checked off a list. I was firm in my belief that he carried immense emotional value just by showing his wife she could trust him to be physically and emotionally present in the most challenging, painful times of their marriage. However, I also recognized the important "do something" nature of his personality and spent some time planning physical tasks and ways he could do something to care for his wife; he named things like making sure she had plenty of tea and water, bringing the children in to play with her when she was at home in bed, and holding her hand while she fell asleep.

With more time with this family, I would have liked to work on additional goals of involving more of Jana's family members than just her husband. I found I was curious, thinking about how Jana's parents would continue to support Tim and his children, even after Jana's death. I thought of these young children, forced to confront the reality of death so young, and wondered how they would make sense of their mother's sudden death and how that understanding would evolve over time. If I were able to continue working with Tim, I would have asked questions like, "What worries you most about raising your children without a living mother?" and directed the conversation into ways that helped promote the family's reliance on getting through struggles together. From our brief conversations, I had learned that Tim and Jana's hometown communities were immensely important to them, and I would have liked to inquire more about what shaped their views of family life through tragedy and how Tim perceived his experience shaping their community members.

Key Learning Points

As Nathaniel Hawthorne wrote, "Time flies over us, but leaves its shadow behind." Time became an essential fact to address in Jana's story of life and death with cancer; it felt like there wasn't enough to fit in all she had left to accomplish as a wife, a mother, a daughter, a community member. She felt this pressure, her husband felt it, and I felt it. Although she had a limited amount of this precious commodity, I am reassured by stories like Jana's because they show that even when time is running out and death stands ready, there is still much life to be had. There are still stories that will be passed down for generations: stories that are infused with loss and sorrow and words like "gone too soon" but also infused with the goodness of a family coming together to be emotionally and physically present during a painful time and in the aftermath. Though death brings sadness, it can also bring a sense of refocusing and purpose to one's days, and this helps contribute to a deep sense of love, trust, and connection to one's family.

REFERENCES

ALS Association (2017). What is ALS? Retrieved October 23, 2017 from www. alsa.org/about-als/what-is-als.html?referrer=https://www.google.com/

Byock, I. (1997). *Dying well: Peace and possibilities at the end of life.* New York, NY: Riverhead Books.

Hargrave, T. D. (1992). *Finishing well: Aging and reparation in the intergenerational family.* New York, NY: Brunner/Mazel.

Ofri, D. (2013). *What doctors feel: How emotions affect the practice of medicine.* Boston, MA: Beacon.

Epilogue

Our journey through this book now comes to a close, and we hope that the stories we have shared provide you with insight and creative strategies, as well as a firm commitment to promote justice and the ethical treatment of all within a family system. First described by Ivan Boszormenyi-Nagy over forty years ago, contextual therapy provides a unique perspective that extends beyond other family therapy models with its focus on systemic justice and relational ethics. The relational factors of love, trust, loyalty, and fairness represent key ingredients that shape the health of relationships and of individuals themselves. To support this point, Goldenthal (1996) wrote:

> It is difficult to find an experienced therapist who would argue with the notion that knowledge of a person's past and present family relationships is crucial to understanding and helping the person, or one who would deny that the issues of loyalty and fairness are central to life and to close relationships. (p. xiii)

Healthy relationships support healthy individuals who are motivated and able to serve their close relationships and broader communities well.

As we have seen through several of the case studies in this book, relationships that are fair, just, and balanced also sustain individuals and families in responding to life's challenges, including acute and chronic illnesses. Although Goldenthal highlighted therapists' awareness of the importance of contextual concepts, we hope that therapists will help illuminate the importance of these concepts in collaboration with other healthcare providers such as physicians, nurses, and care managers. The best way to facilitate this kind of family-centered revolution is to present a cohesive, unified vision from the entire treatment team.

With this book, we aimed to renew and refocus the conversation about this often-forgotten clinical model by highlighting specific ways in which the contextual framework can be used to guide clinical interventions to support biomedical, psychological, social, and spiritual health. We believe one way to increase the appreciation of this clinical model is to clearly apply this framework within healthcare settings and clearly tie contextual constructs to more familiar topics such as motivation for change, barriers to adherence to medical recommendations, and social support systems. Furthermore, more robust research of contextual constructs and their relationships to physical and mental health outcomes is also needed to grow the evidence base for this framework and increase acceptance within the medical community.

One of the most unique aspects of the contextual framework concerns its commitment to the underdog, the person who is likely to be most vulnerable to instances of injustice. In our experience, we have seen countless times when individuals with significant illness either perceive themselves or are perceived by others as weak, vulnerable, and helpless. One thing that makes the contextual model so appropriate for work in healthcare settings is that it allows clinicians to adopt an approach that looks for both vulnerabilities and strengths. Contextually minded clinicians look both for ways in which (1) the patient may be at risk of being mistreated in an unjust way and (2) the patient holds more power and ability than previously thought.

Contextual clinicians can help empower patients to continue contributing to their families and communities in meaningful ways and intervene in the rest of the system to shift boundaries and expectations, restoring fairness and trustworthiness. As we have seen in countless patients' lives, this shift pays out rich rewards. We sincerely hope that you find this, too, in your interactions with patients and their families as you connect on deeper and deeper levels.

REFERENCE

Goldenthal, P. (1996). *Doing contextual therapy: An integrated model for working with individuals, couples, and families.* New York: W.W. Norton.

Index

PGMO 06/13/2018